RETHIN
POSTURE
IN THE MODERN
WORLD

RETHINKING POSTURE IN THE MODERN WORLD

DR. LAWRENCE WOODS

Rethinking Posture in the Modern World
Copyright © 2017 by Lawrence Woods

Disclaimer

Edited by Sinead Moore
Cover illustration by Lawrence Woods

Contents

Foreword

When we are young, our movement patterns are nearly flawless. For the first few years of our life, we utilize movement as a means to explore the complexities of our world. Movement is required to engage the world around us, and so, we quickly learn how to move in complex ways so that we can absorb as much information as possible. We start on our backs, then move to our bellies, and, eventually, we are up on our feet. We are mobile, limber, and free.

Then we step into this modern world and our bodies complacently and unconsciously adapt to our present environment. We are almost perpetually seated from the get-go; car seats; kindergarten, primary and secondary school; 'playdates' that are now spent over computers; video games; college; workplace; television; surfing the web; and so forth. This inevitably leads to the gradual deterioration from primal movements to complacent sedentary postures. Soon the alarm bells of the body start sounding.

There are distinct warning signs that something might be amiss. The first indication that something is wrong is usually some form of pain. You will go to your doctor, who will most likely diagnose you with something like a 'lumbago' (which is a Latin word for back pain), herniation, bulging disc, arthritis or joint degeneration, and so on. Professionals may attempt only to treat the indications rather than the root of the problem. The problem that you are most likely experiencing is a symptom which leads to a predictable breakdown of the body.

We have been conditioned to trust that 'experts' be it a mechanic, priest, teacher, scientist, or doctor have our backs and have a better grasp on our situations than we do. We assume that it is best for them to make decisions on our behalf in their field of expertise. Can this possibly always give us the best outcome? Should these experts be solely accountable for us or do we have any responsibility here?

As a health practitioner, every physical training protocol that this author has witnessed seems to have failed to develop a system that is rooted in human evolution and rudimentary biological capabilities. These models do not fully comprehend the nuances and complexities of human configuration. Lawrence has witnessed a myriad of health and fitness experts who deliver similar narratives about how we can improve our structure and yet, poor posture is still a salient epidemic. We have learned to blindly accept these models as fact without ever utilizing our own critical thinking skills to correct the problems. Lawrence believes that if we continue to adhere to these antiquated models, we are headed down a dangerous path that is saturated with injuries, pain, depression and lack of energy.

How can we possibly shoehorn the human biological system, which is non-lineal, into industry standard treatment protocols, which are generally mechanistic and one-dimensional? Why don't these protocols work? An element seems to be missing here. It appears that most of these techniques are performed in isolation, let's say three hours a week (Pilates, yoga, gym, therapies), and with little consideration of what's going in the remaining one hundred sixty-five.

Perhaps the reason that we continue to adhere to these models is because the healthcare system frowns on deviation from the status quo. In today's healthcare system, each department and individual is assigned a specific role, and they are expected to operate only within the limited scope of their delegated responsibilities. For example, physios work on a muscle, podiatrists work on feet, cardiac surgeons observe the heart, and occupational therapists in the U.S. generally only work on upper extremities. In other words, we have reduced the body to the sum of its parts within a system dedicated to only treating those individual parts, irrespective of the whole. Should anyone deviate from their assigned roles, they are subject to reprimand. Our highly compartmentalized systems have left no room for innovation or challenging ideas, and as such, we operate robotically. What exists in each practitioner beyond their assigned function is of no concern to anyone.

If we look at societies today, we will see that they are becoming increasingly more utilitarian, with people assigned to specific parts that support the good functioning of the overall whole. The person is defined by the extent to which he or she can contribute to the overall scheme or plan. These people make sense only in terms of the overall goal, whether it is the admission of a new patient or the execution of a war.

This is not logical, but is rather palpably reductionist. This line of compartmentalized thinking may be applicable to a project plan, but not to a human being. Logic is a set of rules and principles that is distinctly rational. Logic is rooted in maps and objectives. The individual is not a herd animal that is constrained by labels and directives. The individual is someone who thinks for him or herself. The individual is innovative and can find answers on his or her own and can express and live those answers. He or she is much greater than any institution or linear system and is not designed to succumb to the wants and needs of the establishment.

> *'What is independent of our bodily makeup we are all individually made; each one of us is his or her own self, an individual.' – Rudolf Steiner*

'We just seem to accept everything. Just like in 'The Wizard of Oz,' no one ever pulls the curtain back and asks, 'Why is the artist so interested in conveying this reality?' Wouldn't it be immensely better if we only understood that the power that makes the body, heals it as well?

Herein lies the challenging part. The question 'what should I do?' is typically directed towards persons who are perceived to be experts in their field, whether it be a therapist, doctor or guru. In reality, though, that question should only be directed inward. 'What do I do?' is an inquiry that can only truly be answered by delving deeply into your own critical thinking (why do I have this problem?), and imagination (how am I going to create a solution to this problem?). Although pointers will be given in this manuscript, real solutions can only come from within by utilizing these indicators as ideas for your own personal canvas so that *you* can create your own ways to correct your posture. We believe that the answers to postural deficiencies lie within, but you must do the work to understand them and then take consistent action to alter them.

Most of us have not engaged our imaginations since we were children. If you grew up attending schools or religious organizations, where creativity and inventiveness were stifled, you may have never truly engaged your imagination. It takes time to relearn how to engage one's mind's eye, but it is a necessary endeavour because it is within the complexities of your thoughts that the real solutions to your movement deficiencies lie. Once you get this, you can offload all of your old 'mind' bondage and kick the box wide open.

Lastly, this book was intentionally written in the third person to maintain the objectivity of this material. Lawrence is not a know-it-all or guru, he simply wants to represent his uncommon findings so that you may incorporate a life-style in which he terms an '**actively consciously engaged**' (**ACE**) individual. For example, if you close your eyes right now, can you feel your hands and feet? This is the type of perpetual awareness, engagement, and connection required. It's actually not that difficult to do. Persistence will lead to mastery. Like learning how to drive a car, it starts out with mindful habits which ultimately becomes learned patterns.

1

*Un*common Sense

PHILOSOPHY

You are probably wondering why the author is including a discussion of philosophy in a manuscript about your body's health and well-being. The goal of this book is not to lecture you on how to live your life but to nudge you a little into thinking and making your own decisions about your health, philosophically based on objectivity. The points in this book are simply not being discussed today, even though they are patently obvious. Nobody seems to be paying attention to anything.

Humans, on a consciousl level, have an operating system (think of it as a software system) which is completely external. We humans are different than animals in this regard. For example, if you had a puppy dog raised by a band of gorillas to full maturity, chances are that this dog would think, act, bark, and wag its tail like a dog, since all (non-human) animal's operating system are internal. However, if a human infant was raised by a band of gorillas to full maturity, chances are that this individual would act and think like an ape.* All of our thought processes have been adopted from our parents, educational institutions, clergy, legal society, medical advisors, and so forth. If you step outside your learned operating system, you can find that your own personal intuition and logic will be much more pertinent to you. Much better than any 'wizard' can offer you. However, before embarking down the 'Yellow Brick Road,' one should start any expedition of knowledge with a solid foundation of logic, critical thinking, and philosophy. * http://www.ndtv.com/india-news/the-girl-who-doctors-believe-was-raised-by-monkeys-in-uttar-pradesh-1678691

When most people think of philosophy, they envision great thinkers like Plato, Socrates and Aristotle sitting around, discussing abstract ideas that may appear to be no longer relevant in today's fast-paced and technology-driven world. Truth is, they are still relevant but there is a difference here in that the author is not talking about the *academic* philosophy that dominated those discussions. What Lawrence is referring to is the *application* of philosophical principles in our everyday life.

The basic premise of philosophy is that there is a capacity for error within the human mind and that, because of the fallibility, we must continue to explore and refine it. Philosophy is not something that you can learn in a class or from a book. It's a transformative process. We must continually evaluate our philosophical and value systems in order to be sure that they are aligned with how we are conducting our lives. This premise is still extremely salient as it was in the past.

"Dwell as near as possible to the channel
in which your life flows."
—*Henry David Thoreau*

So you might ask then, how is philosophy relevant to my health? What is the value of incorporating philosophy into my life?

It is really quite simple. Contradictions in your basic philosophical values will facilitate destruction in your life. There is a direct correlation between the amount of chaos and the level of contradictions. If you can perform a realistic inventory of your life and eliminate the contradictions, you will start to observe palpable success in all of your life domains, including your posture and health.

Philosophy has the capacity to take you from confusion and discombobulation to focus and organization. For example, Lawrence worked in conventional medicine for eight years even though he was vehemently opposed to taking drugs. This philosophical conflict created discord in his life and his personal health paid the price. Lawrence is not here to lecture you on right and wrong. What he is advising is to assess whether your life choices are contradicting your core belief system. This is about you discovering your own philosophy and values on health and wellness.

> *"The beginning of a revolution is in*
> *reality the end of a belief."*
> —*Gustave Le Bon*

It must be noted that if you believe that simply thinking positively (an oft-championed tenet by self-help books and gurus) is going to cause improvements to your health, you are going to be sorely disappointed. How you feel about life is simply an ***effect*** of your philosophical foundation, not the ***cause***.

> *Philosophy + Purpose = Cause.*
> *Psychology (Always) = Effect.*

Mental health and physical well-being are the ***effect*** of a solid philosophical foundation. If you try to utilize health and prosperity as the foundation of who you are, then you have things backwards and this will bring you down. In order to achieve a healthy mind and body, it is essential that you begin with clearly defined values, which will eventually buttress sound health and wellness. This distinction is critical and will change your life. Whether aligning your spine or your life's purpose with your philosophical values, this will create focus, which is a critical component to your health. You can only live with purpose if your philosophy and values which are congruent with how you are living your life.

LOGIC

> *"Disease is a disturbed condition,*
> *not a thing or entity."*
> —DD Palmer

Some things have been eating at me for a while and should be eating at you as well. With all the reported advances in terms of 'modern healthcare,' research, consultants, doctors, new technologies, why do we (as a population) keep getting sicker? Why is chronic disease on the rise?

> *"The physician must be able to tell the antecedents,*
> *know the present, and foretell the future—must mediate*
> *these things, and have two special objects*
> *in view with regard to disease, namely,*
> *to do good or to do no harm."*
> —Hippocrates

This quote was uttered by one of the greatest innovators of all time. Was he on to something? Did he know something that we should all know? Hippocrates is often considered by many to be the 'Father of Medicine.' One of his first lessons was related to the obligations that we have as medical professionals, which is simply to '…do no harm.' However, Lawrence wonders to what extent this is an accurate descriptor of today's healthcare system. Although we have made great strides in acute, emergency and traumatic care, we have fallen dangerously short when it comes to chronic degenerative disease and true healthcare. While most health care practitioners and researchers go into their chosen profession with the best of intentions, the fact is, we have insidiously deviated from this notion of 'healthcare' and have adopted a model that is more closely aligned with 'sick care.'

> *"Logical minds, accustomed to being convinced by a chain of somewhat close reasoning, cannot avoid having recourse to this mode of persuasion when addressing crowds, and the inability of their arguments always surprises them."*
> — *Gustave Le Bon (The Crowd)*

With this in mind, let's take a look at what the research tells us about the level of care that we provide today:

Could modern healthcare, which is focused on diagnostic tests, drugs, and surgery, possibly damage more people than it saves? The harms-way of the system may in part due to side effects, whether 'expected' or not. But preventable errors also account for an unequivocally astounding number of deaths.

- According to the most recent research into the cost of medical mistakes in terms of lives lost, 210,000 Americans are killed by preventable hospital errors each year.

  *Journal of Patient Safety; 'A New, Evidence-based Estimate of Patient Harms Associated with Hospital Care'; September 2013: 9(3); 122-128

- When deaths related to diagnostic errors, errors of omission, and failure to follow guidelines are included, the number skyrockets to an estimated 440,000 preventable hospital deaths each year. This is makes medical errors the third-leading cause of death in the US, right after heart disease and cancer.

  *Scientific American September; How Many Die from Medical Mistakes in U.S. Hospitals?; 20, 2013

- According to statistics published in a 2011 Health Grades report, the occurrence rate of medical damage arising in the United States is estimated to be over 40,000 harmful and/or lethal errors daily.

  *HealthGrades 2011 Healthcare Consumerism and Hospital Quality in America Report

- Preventable medical mistakes may account for one-sixth of all deaths that occur in the US annually. To put these numbers into even further perspective, medical mistakes in American hospitals kill four jumbo jets' worth of people each week.

  *The Wall Street Journal; 'How to Stop Hospitals From Killing Us'; September 21, 2012

- Out of the 783,936 annual deaths from conventional medicine mistakes, approximately 106,000 of those are the result of prescription drug use.

  *Null, G PHD. (2011). Death by Medicine. Mount Jackson, VA: Praktikos Books.

- Prescription drugs are now killing far more people than illegal drugs, and while most major causes of preventable deaths are declining, those from prescription drug use are increasing, an analysis of recently released data from the U.S. Centers for Disease Control and Prevention (CDC) by the Los Angeles Times revealed.

  *Los Angeles Times September 17, 2011

It is difficult to know the exact numbers of casualties from these studies. However, we can deduce that these reports should be taken as a wake-up call and perhaps we can think more critically when it comes to our health.

Let's pause here for a minute and discuss the meaning of this nebulous term, 'health.' What is it and what exactly does it mean? Does it mean feeling good? Does it simply mean the absence of 'symptoms?' According to Dorland's Medical Dictionary, 'health is a state of optimal physical, mental and social well-being, and not merely the absence of disease and symptoms.' Most of us tend to base our characterization on the second part of this definition and wholly neglect the first part, which refers to optimal functioning.

What does optimal mean? It means operating at 100%. How can we get our bodies to this optimal state? Well, that takes work. You must first take care of the most fundamental needs of the body, which means nourishing it with clean food, water, optimal oxygenation (clean air, exercise) and getting adequate sleep. If you remove any of these components you may cease to exist. Nevertheless, if they are interfered with on a qualitative or quantitative level, chances are that you are going to impede with your health potential.

Conversely in saying this, these constituents (proper food, water, oxygenation, sleep) are not the complete picture. There is another factor of health that is of equal importance and statistically no one ever even thinks about it. This component is your **structure**.

The late Thomas Edison stated:

"The doctor of the future will give no medicine, but will interest his patients in the care of the human frame (spine), in diet and in the cause and prevention of disease."

Hippocrates stated:

"Get knowledge of the spine, for this is the requisite for many diseases."

We now have two prominent historical figures who recognized the inextricable link between the 'health' and its connection with the spine. The spine is critically important because it is the source of the spinal nerves, which, in tandem with the spinal cord, control and coordinate the functions of the human body. When there is a mechanical deficiency, it can impact the transmission of the electric signal the nerve is carrying to the muscle, organ or tissue. This can create an imbalance and dissension within the body and can give rise to any number of maladies. A purpose of this book is to make the connection between your structure and your health using critical thinking and logic.

2

The Foundation

Growing up as a youngster in New Jersey, the author always wanted to be a superhero. He wanted to save the planet from sickness and disease. On a more personal level, he wanted to save his younger brother (Brian) who was ill from the age of four and lived to the age of twenty-nine.

On his brother's deathbed, he asked a question that would eventually become the driving force behind his life's work. He wanted to know why there seemed to be a disproportionate amount of time and effort dedicated to working with those who were ill versus those who were healthy. Why, he wondered, weren't comparable resources being dedicated to understanding the habits of those who were healthy?

With this question in mind, he came up with a plan. Lawrence decided to set off and interview anyone who had lived to 90+ years and who was still in reasonably good health. He believed that the answers that he sought would reveal themselves in these interviews. Lawrence travelled everywhere to interview seemingly 'healthy' people. He evaluated habits like their mental health, nutrition, sleep and exercise regimens.

Of course, all of these elements are critically important for sustained health. However, he could not make the determination that there was a definitive connection between any single element (taken in isolation) and health endurance. Lawrence is sure that you know, as well as he does, that many people who do all the 'right things' can still succumb to chronic disease.

It's reasonable to think of what's essential for sustained life…things such as clean food, water, exercise, and plenty of rest should also be the essential components to sustained health. Though this seems logical, in his years and years of research, he couldn't find a definitive relationship between these life-sustaining components and overall health.

He felt defeated. He began believing that maybe we come into our bodies with a predetermined number of healthy days, and that sickness and death were inevitable. However, many years later, after having already given up on Brian's quest, he made a discovery that was a massive blind spot which he never thought of.

Lawrence was having a casual conversation with a dear old friend (Paul), who was in his mid-80s at the time, and whom he never thought to interview for his little study, because he didn't fit his algorithm. Paul lived an active life. He was a rebel who didn't live by the rules. Paul was kind of agnostic towards 'modern health care.' In fact, he's never really been to a doctor apart from a few stitches here and there. Lawrence asked Paul, 'What's your secret staying so young and full of energy and in great shape?' He replied, 'I don't have any. No secrets. My diet, sleep, and exercise are kind of sporadic. You know me Lawrence, I'm always on the go, just can't sit still.' In that moment, in the middle of this casual conversation, the penny dropped.

Let's take a moment to analyze this connection that is going to change your life. In order to do so and to fully comprehend the magnitude of Paul's words, we must first take a step back before you became you.

BACK TO THE BEGINNING…

Way, way back, two half cells had a fortuitous meeting and started to multiply. After about 8 weeks, these cells developed a first organ. Can you guess what the first organ was? Many assume that it is the heart or the skeleton, but they are incorrect. The first organ formed is the brain and the spinal cord (Central Nervous System – CNS). Subsequently to the formation of the control system, you then develop body parts such as the lungs, kidneys and skeleton.

For everything to work correctly, you need a nerve supply from the brain and spinal cord. It is the electrical energy that courses through our body that differentiates us from corpses. Anatomically, in fact, we are identical to corpses. The differentiating factor is the electricity.

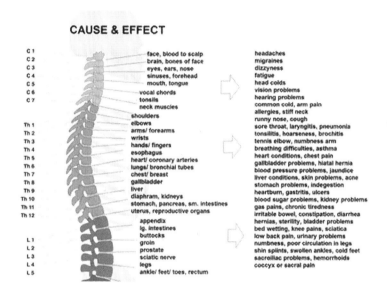

The primary protectors of your central nervous system are the skull, twenty four vertebrae and the pelvis. In between each of these spinal segments is a pair of spinal nerves that bring messages from the brain to the individual parts of the body. Different segments are responsible for the transmission of messages to different parts of the body. The general rule of thumb is that the higher segments communicate with the upper portion of the body, while the lower segments communicate with the lower portion of the body.

The way the body works is complex yet simple. A message begins in the brain, travels down the spinal cord to a specific spinal nerve, which then initiates a particular action within. Then, when the process is complete, a message travels back through that nerve, up the spinal cord and into the brain, and communicates whether or not that action was completely successfully.

But what happens if that communication is impeded in some way by bad posture thus causing a change in the curvature or rotation of the spine?

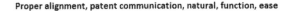

Proper alignment, patent communication, natural, function, ease

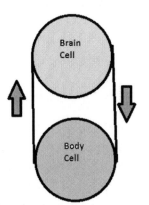

The tissue cell sends impulses to the brain communicating what it needs for proper function

Brain cell responds by coordinating the various systems of the body to supply what is demanded from the body

The simple analogy of the safety pin may help you internalize the relationship between the spine and overall health. When the body is functioning correctly, there is reciprocal communication between the brain and every cell, tissue and organ in the body. Both paths are uninterrupted, just like a closed safety pin. Problems arise when there is a disruption in either of these communication paths. In this case, the safety pin is open (where it is no longer functioning optimally) and the body slips into a state of disease.

Mis-**alignment,** *mis*-**communication,** *un*-**natural,** *mal*-**function,** *dis*-**ease**

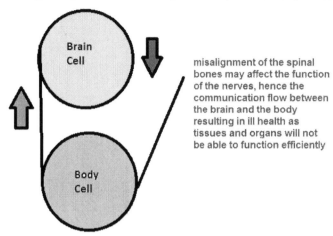

misalignment of the spinal bones may affect the function of the nerves, hence the communication flow between the brain and the body resulting in ill health as tissues and organs will not be able to function efficiently

A subluxation is a condition that manifests when a spinal bone is misaligned in relation to the one above or the one below and exerts pressure on the nerve in between them. You can have a single subluxation or multiple ones at a time. At the University of Colorado in the early 1970s, Professor Chung-Ha Suh conducted a research project that studied the effects of compression on spinal nerve roots*. He found that even minuscule amounts of pressure on a nerve root (10mm Hg, equal to a feather falling on your hand) could result in up to a 50 percent decrease in the capacity of that nerve to transmit electricity. The end result is disrupted communication to the part of the body that the nerve innervates, which can dramatically reduce function.

Solid posture is the foundation upon which everything else related to your health should be built. For some reason though, structural integrity is almost never considered to be a critical component of our health. The role that the back and spinal cord play in our overall health and vitality deserves much more attention than it is currently afforded in our healthcare system. Keeping the back healthy isn't just important in order to prevent back pain, it is critical to your longevity.

* Dr. Chung-Ha Suh, Seth Sharpless, Ph.D., Marvin Luttges, Ph.D. ; University of Colorado Project; 1970

3

Connection between Posture and Health Using Critical Thinking and Logic

Why is good posture so important? Most of us are lucky enough to be born with a good spine. But what happens to our spines as we age and what causes deterioration? Without knowing anything about you, if you are reading this book, chances are that you most likely have a posture problem. You are not alone. It appears that this condition is ubiquitous to just about everyone in the Western world. The trouble isn't just that slumped shoulders make you resemble the Hunchback of Notre Dame. Over time, your poor posture takes a tremendous toll on your spine, shoulders, hips, knees and, eventually, your health. In fact, it can cause a cascade of structural flaws that result in acute problems, such as joint pain throughout your body, reduced flexibility and compromised muscles, and, ultimately, systemic health problems.

On a local level, when a spinal bone (vertebrae) moves out of its ideal position (subluxation) and causes irritation on spinal nerves (which protrude from between the bones of the spine), this may cause a malfunction and interference with the signaling between your brain and body. An important element of this book is to guide you in restoring and maintaining the spinal bones (vertebrae) back to their idyllic position, thus reducing or eliminating nerve pressure, and allowing all of the parts of the body to work synchronously.

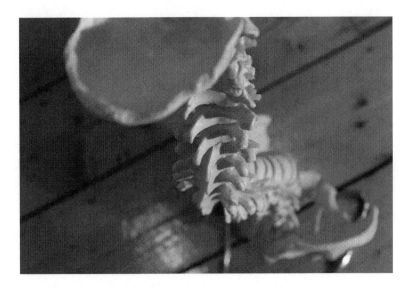

So when we look at nerve supply, if your brain stops working, can you exist? If your posture is imbalanced and your spinal bones are misaligned, do you think it is possible to achieve optimal health, even if you are addressing the other essential intangibles? Absolutely not! One must have a nervous system that is operating unimpeded, so that all parts of the body are, in turn, functioning without interference.

'Subluxations are very real. We have documented it to the extent that no one can dispute their existence. Vertebral Subluxations change the entire health of the body by causing structural dysfunction of the spine and nerve interference. The weight of a quarter on a spinal nerve will decrease nerve transmission by as much as 60 percent.'
—Chang Ha Suh, PhD

As you now can recall, the spine (or backbone), as well as the brain, are the primary components of the central nervous system (CNS). The central nervous system is responsible for the functioning of every single cell, tissue and organ in the human body.

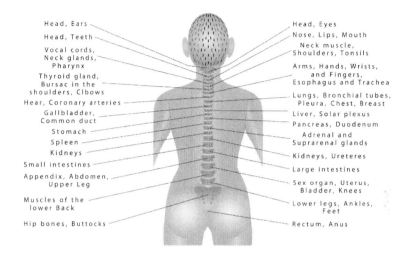

The peripheral nervous system (PNS) refers to the parts of the nervous system outside of the brain and spinal cord. This includes all of the nerves and cells. The PNS is responsible for the transmission of signals between the central nervous system and the rest of the human body. Unlike the spinal cord, the PNS is not encased in bone. Because of this, it is highly susceptible to damage and interference. This system must be adequately cared for, or else our overall health may be at risk.

As indicated previously, if the structure and alignment of the spine is altered or if there is damage to the surrounding and connecting tissues, the impact could be catastrophic. Damage to the peripheral nervous system can lead to limitations in mobility, weakened immunity to diseases, and organ deterioration. One study* conducted by researchers at the University of Pennsylvania indicated that there was 100% correspondence between the slight curvatures in the spine and diseases of the internal organs as demonstrated of 75 human and 72 cat cadavers:

Heart Disease – All twenty cases with heart and pericardium conditions had the upper five thoracic vertebrae misaligned (T1-T5).

Lung Disease – All twenty-six cases of lung disease has spinal misalignments in the upper thoracic area.

Stomach Disease – All nine cases of stomach disease had spinal misalignment in the mid-thoracic (T5-T9) area.

Liver Disease – All thirteen cases of liver disease had misalignments in the mid-thoracic area (T5-T9).

Gallbladder – All five cases with gallstone disease had spinal misalignments in the mid-thoracic area (T5-T9).

Pancreas – All three cases with pancreas disease had spinal misalignments in the mid-thoracic area (T5-T9).

Spleen – All eleven cases with spleen disease had spinal misalignments in the mid-thoracic area (T5-T9).

Kidney – All seventeen cases with kidney disease were out of alignment in the lower thoracic area (T10-T12).

Prostate and Bladder Disease – All eight cases with prostate disease had the lumbar vertebrae misaligned.

Uterus – Two cases with uterine conditions had the second lumbar misaligned.

This just reiterates the importance of the spine in maintaining homeostatic balance in the body and overall health.

* Winsor H. Sympathetic Segmental Disturbances—II. The evidences of the association, in dissected cadavers, of visceral disease with vertebrae deformities of the same sympathetic segments; Medical Times, November 1921; 49:267-271

"The quality of healing is directly proportional to the functional capability of the central nervous system to send and receive nerve messages."
—Janson Edwards, MD. PhD

Since nerve interference (subluxation) affects the transmission of signals to various parts of the body, it simultaneously effects and creates changes to various components and this is what manifests physically as a result of bad posture.

LET'S LOOK AT WHAT IS INVOLVED WHEN SPINAL BONES MISALIGN

The Bone (Osseous) Component – this primary component experiences the changes brought about by vertebral subluxation. Due to the dislocation of some of the vertebral bones, degeneration is more prone to happen. Rapid deterioration of bones is expected and posture is greatly affected.

The Nerve Component – this is the recipient of the changes that happen in the bone component. Bones push the nerves, creating pressure and affecting their complex functions. It is worth noting that nerves are very delicate parts of our body. Thus, they are very vulnerable to sudden increases in pressure and slight disturbances.

The Muscle Tissue – since muscles hold the vertebrae in place, they are also affected by any changes caused by subluxation. In addition, nerves control the activities of muscles. Thus, any changes that nerves experience have an equivalent change in the muscle component. The combination of nerve and muscle components is more commonly known as myopathology.

The Soft Tissue Component – it has been established in the previous chapters that soft tissues like ligaments and tendons surround the vertebrae and are therefore affected by any changes that they undergo. Soft tissue injuries are also the most common effect of bad posture such as sitting. Muscles, tendons and ligaments are also damaged during exercise and sporty activities conducted with bad posture. Even basic lifting, reaching for something and bending can cause sudden trauma or twist soft tissues, and that, in turn, can damage these tissues.

The Biochemical Component – this is the result of all the changes in the other components of your body. Naturally, our body reacts to any changes that it detects as a coping mechanism. With any interference in the nerve supply affecting the organs and glands, homeostasis goes out the window.

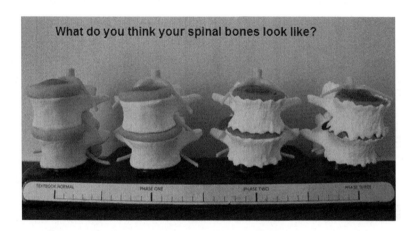

COMMON SYMPTOMS/ DISORDERS FROM SPINAL MISALIGNMENT:

While there are many different diagnoses for back disorders, most of these problems share a singular point of origin: degenerative changes in the vertebrae of the spine and in the intervertebral discs. These are often subclinical and unnoticeable changes which herald diagnosable conditions.

Low Back Pain – Low back pain is one of the most common health complaints in the world. Nearly everyone gets back pain at some point in their life.* There are many different types of pain. *Acute* back pain is defined as severe but lasting a short period of time. *Chronic* back pain usually occurs every day. It can be severe, but may be characterized as mild, deep, achy, burning, or electric-like. Back pain that migrates into another part of the body, such as the leg may be considered radicular pain (principally when it radiates below the knee). This scenario is commonly called a lumbar radiculopathy. Approximately one fourth of all US adults reported having low back pain thus making it the leading contributor to missed work.**

*A systemic review and metasynthesis of the impact of low back pain and people's lives; BMC Musculoskelet Disord.; 2014;15:50

**A systemic review of the global prevalence of low back pain; Arthritis Rheum. 2012;64(6);2028-2037

Degenerative Joint Disease (DJD) – One of the most debilitating effects of these micro-changes is degenerative joint and disc disease. Joint and disc disease is the precursor to many incapacitating back conditions, osteoarthritis of the spine, facet joint disorders, and spinal stenosis (a painful and sometimes devastating condition, which involves a narrowing of the spinal canal).

If you have never had a disc problem, then you might presume that degenerative disc disease doesn't have much relevance in your life. Unfortunately, that might not be the case. The asymptomatic micro-changes associated with degenerative disc disease are much more common than most people realize. MRI studies of healthy people, without any presenting symptoms of back problems, have shown that, among patients from 20 years old to 40, one in three showed degenerative decompensation in the lumbar spine. In people aged 40 to 60, that number increases to almost six out of ten. In individuals aged 60-80, almost 80% showed some degree of disc degeneration.*

* http://www.iowasource.com/health/2009_11_spine.html

Joint and disc degeneration is a progressive, degenerative condition, which worsens with age. The more advanced the deterioration of the disc, the greater the likelihood that the degeneration will spread to other parts of the spine. Degenerative disc disease is so common, in fact, that many doctors perceive it as an inevitable by-product of old age.

Osteoarthritis is considered a form of degenerative joint disease because it occurs when the cartilage that normally surrounds and protects the joints wears away. When the cartilage is worn away, bones rub against one another, thus causing swelling and pain.

Most of us will claim that arthritis is a disease of aging people. However, bad posture can cause arthritis even within a younger demographic. Our spine cartilage often gets damaged easily due to incorrect posture, poor body positioning during physical activities, and sedentary lifestyles. Maintaining a good posture is not just about looking physically good. We may not know it, but there are threats to our health that can be prevented by maintaining a straight spine.

Again, these degenerative changes have a much more profound impact on the body through nerve interference. Subtle structural alterations put pressure on the delicate, infinitesimal nerve filaments which flow through the spinal cord. When the nerve flow is impeded, organs or body parts may not receive the messages they need in order to maintain their function. The effect is the equivalent of stepping on a water hose and disrupting the flow of water to your garden. If there are multiple distortional patterns, this disruption may be widespread and communication may be compromised across the body. This subsequently can impact the overall health of the body.

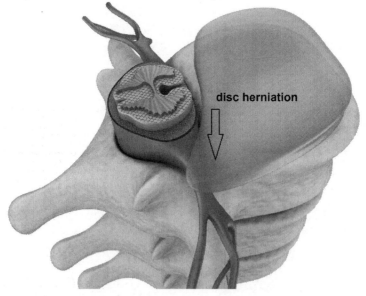

disc herniation

Disc herniation, disc protrusion and 'slipped discs'- are sometimes used as interchangeable terms, especially among healthcare professionals. To add some clarity here, disc herniation is typically an additional by-product of a previously existing disc protrusion. Disc herniation is usually due to degeneration caused by improper sitting, lifting or straining. Subluxations ultimately lead to disc herniation (also known as a slipped disc) which is a disorder affecting the spine in which a tear in the external fibrous layer of the spinal disc that allows the soft, central portion to bulge outside the injured external layers. This is a condition in which the outermost layers of the fibrous ring of the disc are still intact, but can bulge and create small tears when under pressure. These tears in the outer disc layers can produce the discharge of inflammatory chemical mediators, which could cause severe pain, even in the absence of nerve root compression.

'**Text neck**' is now a worldwide epidemic affecting millions of people of all ages and from all walks of life, and it is caused by a pervasive overuse of handheld mobile technology, resulting in potentially permanent damaging physical conditions of the body.

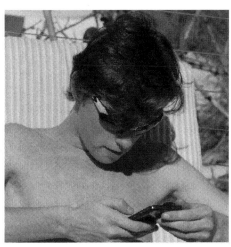

For every inch (2.54cm) of forward head position caompared to a neutral position, the weight of the head increases by 10 pounds (4.5kg) on the spine. This forward head position has been linked to many health problems, including decreased lung capacity, altered blood pressure, headaches and digestive issues.
-Kapandji; Physiology of Joints; Vol 3

Another point here is the connection between slouched behaviour with a forward head translation (text neck posture) and depression.

Depressed people often have altered postures. If you force them out of that posture, they may become less depressed. The posture we adopt when we're over those phones mirrors a depressed person's posture. It begs the question, logically, where are we going with these problems? Do we really need to wait 10-15 years to see a new study that examines the carnage of all of this?

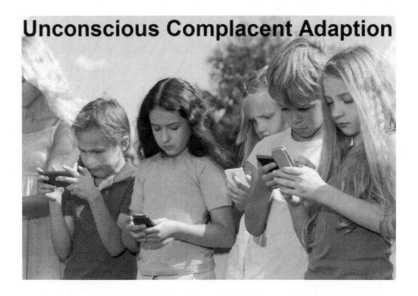

Unconscious Complacent Adaption

A study found that when your spine is in neutral position, the head weighs about 10-12 pounds. At 15 degrees [forward], the neck sees 27 pounds. At 45 degrees, it sees 49 pounds, and at 60 degrees, it's 60 pounds. When you have such aggressive stressors on the neck, you get wear and tear on the spine. You can develop tears within the disc or even get a slipped or herniated disc.' In other words, it is equivalent to 60 pounds of pressure stressing the muscles and nerves that are meant to handle only around 10 pounds of pressure, which, in time, will do a lot of destruction. Think about what this is doing to our children?

* 'Text neck' is becoming an epidemic and could wreck your spine'. The Washington Post. 20 November 2014.

Of the approximately 7.5 billion people on this planet, over 4.77 billion have mobile phones. Even though texting has become the dominant form of communication, 'text neck' is not just restricted to the results of texting and overemployment of cell phones. Most individuals spend innumerable hours daily stooped over a plethora of handheld gadgets, including tablets, media players, etc. one billion text messages are sent every month worldwide Americans spend almost 5 hours per day on their phone. Americans check their phones 8 billion times a day (46 times a day per phone). *journals.plos.org; Time 12/15/2015

Sciatica – sciatic neuritis or lumbar radiculopathy is characterised by extreme pain sensed from the lower back going down to the legs. This condition is usually instigated by spinal disc herniation that presses on one of the lumbar nerves causing severe pain, which is usually aggravated when sitting. The pressing of lumbar nerves is brought about by bad posture that has caused spinal discs to protrude. This is a very serious disease since it can lead to permanent nerve and tissue damage if not addressed immediately.

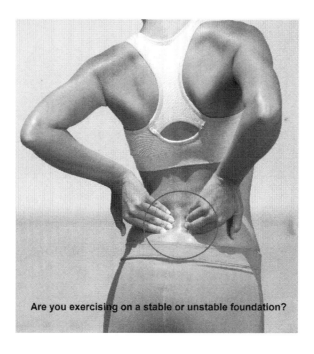

Are you exercising on a stable or unstable foundation?

Treatment for sciatica neuritis can be either surgical or non-surgical. Non-surgical medical procedures are done just to dismiss the pain. However, this does not address the root cause of the problem. These treatments include the application of hot/cold compresses, pain reliever medication and epidural steroid injections for sciatica. Alternative non-medical or non-surgical sciatica treatments are now gaining popularity, as they offer safer treatments with long-lasting effects. Most patients with sciatica now undergo spinal adjustments, non-surgical spinal decompression (Lawrence's favorite!), deep tissue laser therapy, acu-puncture and massage therapy. However, there is no better way to prevent sciatica other than maintaining proper and good posture.

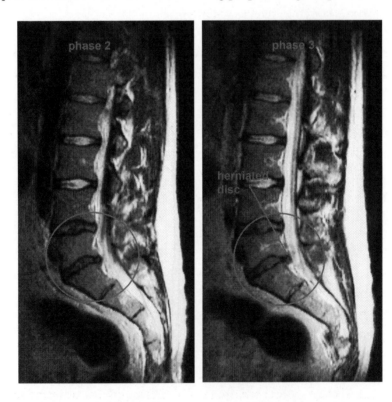

Are distortional patterns an issue for you? Absolutely. Everyone suf-fers, to a certain extent, from distortional patterns in the soft tissues or bones. It is a natural by-product of stress, whether it be mental, physical or chemical. However, whether or not you experience symptoms as a result of these distortions is completely contingent on the extent to which you take actionable steps to mitigate their influence, especially as you age.

Headaches – There are a plethora of reasons for headaches that go way outside the scope of this book. One root cause of many headache sufferers' pain may not in the head but in the spine of the neck (cervical spine). A recent study of more than 5,000 headache sufferers determined that about 40 percent of incidences start from misaligned spinal bones (vertebrae) of the neck (cervical spine).*

   *Wien Med Wochenschr; 1994;144:102-8

Chronic Conditions Usually Stem from Physical, Chemical, and Emotional Causes:

Physical causes are related to physical aspects we deal with on a day to day basis including bad posture, poor sitting techniques, weak or imbalanced spinal musculature, repetitive motions, and acute trauma.

- **POOR POSTURE – sitting at desk, driving, overuse of media technology**
- birth trauma
- childhood falls
- broken bones
- sports injuries
- car accidents
- surgeries
- heavy lifting

Chemical causes are related to chemicals and toxins that are introduced into our body. These chemicals come from the foods we ingest, the liquids we drink, and the air we breathe. Sometimes they are intentional such as through drug or alcohol abuse. Other times they are unintentional such as poor diet and nutrition. Chemicals that are harmful decrease the body's ability to function and impedes our ability to deal with both internal and external stresses.

- **Chemicals in food, water, air, environment**
- Toxic ingredients in medications/vaccines
- smoking
- alcohol abuse
- caffeine overuse
- mother given drugs during pregnancy

Emotional causes pertain to stress. Medical research has proven that emotional stress effects physical health. When stress grows to extreme levels and stress management isn't working well, the body responds with possibly tightened muscles, spinal misalignment, and cessation of normality in its everyday function. This malfunction can affect the immune system, which leads to injury and disease.

- job stress
- financial worries
- bad relationship
- divorce
- abuse
- personal stress
- loss of a loved one

Many of the stresses mentioned here go beyond the scope of this book. However, in saying this, simple changes outlined in the following chapters can have a major impact on your structure and health. But, you must create conditions in your life that are optimal for achieving health. It's that simple. You reap what you sow. If you place a seed in poor soil and neglect it, the plant that grows will be weak, small, shriveled and vulnerable to disease. However, if you provide that same seed the appropriate nourishment, it will yield a strong, healthy and productive plant. How are you tending your own seeds (cells), and how will you care for them in the future?

This brings us back to Paul again, whose longevity was likely supported by a balanced body that he had maintained for decades. Can you imagine if Paul wasn't so active? What if he sat for a living? How do you think his health would have turned out and would he had been able to maintain this balance over so many years?* If you recall Lawrence's conversation with Paul, he told Lawrence that he doesn't sit much. On memory, this may have been the common thread between all of Lawrence's interviewees that he had been searching for. **They didn't sit!** Prolonged sitting causes breakdown in the communication between the central nervous system and the body. This breakdown can subsequently leave the body vulnerable to all sorts of mechanical errors. It is similar to a rock getting lodged in a hose that is watering a garden. This obstruction will deprive the plants of the necessary nutrients that they need to survive, just as sitting for extended periods of time impedes the communicative capacities of the body.

The evidence to support this is overwhelming. There are 10,000+ publications that have found that prolonged sitting can be extremely detri-mental to your overall health. Sitting down too much actively promotes dozens of chronic diseases including obesity, type 2 diabetes, heart disease, cancer, and depression. Now that you understand the impact that a sedentary lifestyle can have on the internal functions, it makes perfect sense that prolonged sitting might contribute to the development of these ailments.

When you sit, you bend your spine, which can initiate the pattern of breakdown that signals pain. Your doctor will likely provide you options to mitigate the pain, but they won't provide you solutions for correcting the problem. The problem is not the pain, but rather a dysfunctional movement pattern which has catalyzed communication breakdown in the body.

---

*Other considerations with Paul might be that his diet is simple (mostly local) and he is a relatively happy guy.

4

It's All Connected

By now, you should rudimentary connection between the communication with the brain and the body by means of the nervous system. However, the brain and nervous system does not actually give us the full picture on how the body works. If we dig down a little deeper, we will find that there are other parallel systems that explain the vast networks and communications of the body. These systems are the endocrine and collagen systems.

So, if we go to a more intrinsic level, the brain and spinal cord are inextricably linked to the body's health capacities because they control your body's chemistry. It is your body's chemistry that determines how much energy you have, how well you sleep, your moods, and how well you get along with others.

Let's take a look at the role of chemistry in your body. As you're reading this, you are likely sitting down, and your heart is beating normally. Now suppose that, all of a sudden, the building caught on fire and you needed to escape quickly. If your body chemistry doesn't change in this moment, you will be rendered incapacitated and unable to generate the requisite energy to flee.

There are small glands in the body called adrenal glands, and they are responsible for the production of adrenaline. For you to generate the required energy to escape the fire, you have to have adrenaline pumped into your bloodstream. If you don't, you will lack the energy, power and speed to survive. Virtually everything that you do requires a manipulation of your body's chemistry, even something as innocuous as falling asleep.

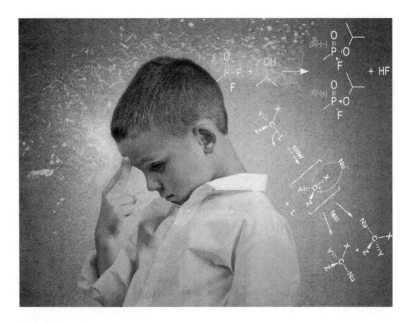

Your body chemistry influences many things. It is directly correlated to your capacity to resist disease. If you breathe in pollen during the summertime, your body responds by making a chemical called histamine. Now, if your body is producing appropriate levels of histamine, you will likely not have a reaction to the pollen. If the person's body next to you is producing too much histamine, they might experience a runny nose and watery eyes, and might say something like, 'the pollen is making me sick.' In reality, it is not the pollen that is making you sick, but rather your imbalanced body chemistry, which does not have the capacity to produce appropriate levels of histamine.

*Did you know that your sense of humor is
controlled by chemistry?*

When your chemistry is out of balance, you will never achieve your full potential. There are trillions of cells in your body, and each one is a chemical factory. They produce chemicals that are crucial to your survival. If your chemistry is properly balanced, you are as strong as a horse; if it is out of balance, you may be susceptible to all sorts of maladies.

So what does all of this have to do with your brain and spinal cord? In order for you to produce the correct chemicals at the appropriate time, there has to be a master control system that monitors the entire body. For example, how does your heart know exactly how much activity your legs are producing? Fortunately, your body comes equipped with a central monitoring system that can process and synthesize copious amounts of information almost instantaneously: the brain and spinal cord.

In 1910, D.D. Palmer wrote:

'Physiologists divide nerve-fibers, which form the nerves, into two classes, afferent and efferent. Impressions are made on the peripheral afferent fiber-endings; these create sensations which are transmitted to the center of the nervous system. Efferent nerve-fibers carry impulses out from the center to their endings. Most of these go to muscles and are therefore called motor impulses; some are secretory and enter glands; a portion are inhibitory their function being to restrain secretion. Thus, nerves carry impulses outward and sensations inward. The activity of these nerves, or rather their fibers, may become excited or allayed by impingement, the result being a modification of functioning — too much or not enough action — which is dis-ease.'

Another immense communication network (which is distinct from the endocrine or nervous systems) is a new field of research is called the collagen (biophotonic) system. Although the biophotonic model is in its infancy, it will be discussed here because it may give us clues on a deeper level how the body works and also why things go wrong. This research is new but the concept is ancient. If you ever want to learn something new and cutting edge, read a very old book!

If you visit any maternity ward (in this modern world), you will most likely find a unit with newborns under a blue light. If you ask any of the staff who work at one of these facilities, 'what are these blue lights for?' You might get an explanation that the lights reduce the yellowing of the skin which is caused by excessive amounts of bile pigments in blood tissues. However, if you do a cursorily search on this subject you may find that the first deliberate use of this type of light as a form of medical treatment can be traced back around 1400 BC to 600 BC India Ayurveda (Indian traditional medicine). They achieved this by using blue quartz and sunlight. These ancients somehow made the connection that the frequency of blue light had a profound healing effect on the cells of the liver.

Our body is composed of trillions of cells, which are the fundamental building blocks of a human body. A group of cells that performs similar functions is referred to as a tissue. The human body, as complex as it is, is made up of 4 major classifications of tissues, namely the epithelial, muscle, nervous and connective tissues.

Connective tissues play an essential role in the human body. They fill in the spaces between various organs and tissues to facilitate cohesion. Furthermore, they help build the structural and metabolic support for other organs and tissues. The base configuration of connective tissue has a liquid-crystallinity structure, which makes it conductive to bioelectric energy. The meninges, for example, is made up of connective tissues in our central nervous system that cover the brain and the spinal column.

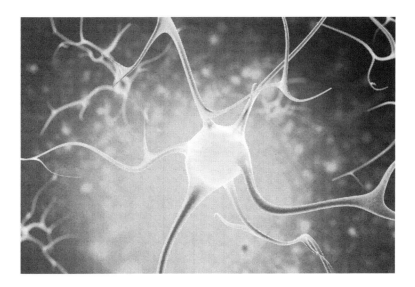

Bioelectric communication research via connective tissue was pioneered by Fritz-Albert Popp (Vibrational Medicine)*. Russian scientist Pjotr Garjajev managed to identify the communicative capacities of connective tissue in the form of ultraviolet photons or, more precisely, biophotons. Biophotons are light emissions from all living organisms. Following the work of Popp and Garjajev, scientists around the globe have begun to consider that our body's communication system might be a complex network of frequency and resonance.

* Popp, F. A., Li, K., Gu. Q. (1992) Recent advances in biophoton research and its application, World scientific, 1-18.

** Russian DNA Research; www.psychicchildren.co.uk/4-3-RussianDNAResearch.html

Did you know that out of the 100 trillion cells in your body, each cell has over 100,000 biochemical reactions per second, all of which must be carefully timed and sequenced with each other? The 'mechanical' concept whereby molecules bump into each other by chance and fit together like a lock and key, or by changing shape in order to come together and form chemical reactions must no longer hold any validity. It's just too slow to explain cell-to-cell communication for 100,000 biochemical reactions per second multiplied by 100,000,000,000 cells!

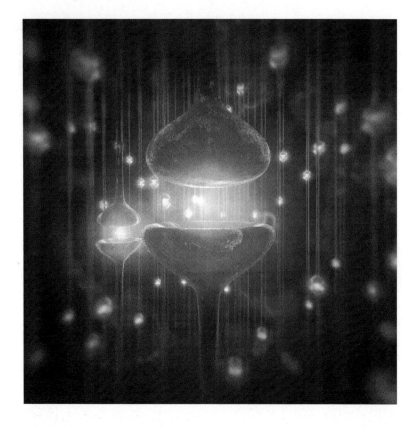

Scientists are starting to concede that this cellular dance is not random at all, but rather controlled by biophotons. Dr. Popp, who proved the existence of the biophoton field in 1974, believes that these types of 'biophoton emissions' are responsible for transferring information throughout your entire body. Coincidentally, the term 'subluxation' was first coined in the late 1800's by D.D. Palmer*, meaning: less light in the brain-to-cell communication.

* Ancestry of Daniel David Palmer". Wargs.com. October 20, 1913

Your body actually emits light on a daily basis, primarily through your connective tissue, in concentrations that rise and fall with your body clock and the rhythmic fluctuations of your metabolism. Most people cannot detect the light because it is 1,000 times less intense than levels that can be seen with the naked eye. Some believe they are able to see this emitted light or 'aura' and some can even distinguish colours in it. Fritz Albert Popp was the first to suggest that this light must be coming, at least in part, from the foods we eat. When we eat plant foods, the light waves, or biophotons, in the plants are taken in and stored by your body. The more light a food is able to store, the more nutritious it is. Naturally grown fresh vegetables, for example, and sun-ripened fruits are rich in light energy. The ability to store biophotons is, therefore, a measure of the quality of our food.

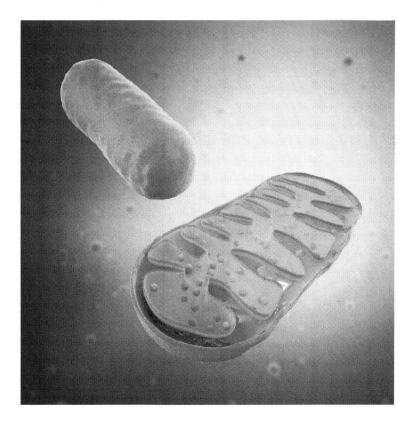

Biophotons are the smallest physical units of light which are stored in and used by all living things. The purpose of these biophotons is much more significant than many have previously thought. It turns out they may very well be in charge of virtually every biochemical reaction that occurs in your body – including supporting your body's ability to heal.*

"The use of light as a natural form of energy from nature actually activates the normal biochemistry of the cell so that the cell tends to take from it what it needs."
— *Dr. Harry Whelan, MD*

The research done by Popp also showed that the light emissions of healthy people follow a set biological rhythm for day and night, as though they are coupled to biorhythms of the earth as well. However, in his studies, the light emissions from diseased patients, such as those with cancer, had no such rhythms and appeared scrambled, which suggests that their cells were no longer communicating efficiently.*

* Mondovista; Is DNA the Next Internet?; Dan Eden 2010

It may be understood that cancer-causing chemicals alter your body's biophoton emissions, interrupting cellular communications.

Have ever noticed that animals have a spinal column is horizontal or parallel to the surface of the earth and that man is perpendicular or vertical to the surface of the earth? There are fields on this earth (just look at any compass).* Look into perpendicular lines of force on the planet and how some researchers believe that there is a connection these lines of force and the spine, brain and the biophotinic system.**

*The exception here is birds which generally stand at 36 degrees which is a diagonal of a cube. (Pythagoras)

**More insight on this topic on www.EricDollard.com, www.nobelprize.org/nobel_prizes /physics/laureates/1906/thomson-bio.html

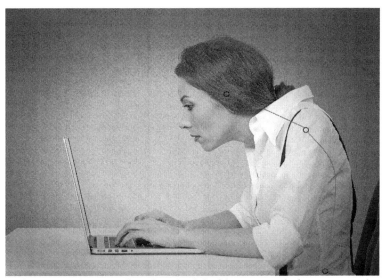

when your muscles contract for prolonged periods of time, your muscles become ropey and adhesions which creates postural disturbances, disc degeneration and overstated spinal curves

WHAT DOES THE BIOPHOTONIC SYSTEM HAVE TO DO WITH POSTURE?

The connective tissues of your lungs and diaphragm are connected to your spine, digestive tract, liver, heart, pelvis, legs, feet, arms, hands, head, etc. The main point here is that connective tissue is connected! This connective tissue shrinks or tightens in response to any form of stress, be it physical, chemical or, most importantly, mental stress. This tightening can detrimentally impact the communicative capacities of your connective tissues.

When your posture contracts for prolonged periods of time, pressure through the crystalline structure signals specialized cells (within the connective tissue) to create more fiber. This causes overlapping fascia sheaths (layers of connective tissue) to become tacky and cement to each other, similar to Velcro. This causes terrible knots or ropiness in your muscles. For example, a forward-head-translation posture can cause chronic tension, which can subsequently cause the fascia sheaths around the involved muscles to form adhesion. This adhesion will likely hinder range-of-motion and make it difficult to stretch out. This may eventually lead to disc degeneration and the configuration of an overstated spinal curvature known as Dowager's hump. Another and perhaps graver problem is that the cell-to-cell communication of the biophotons becomes hindered.

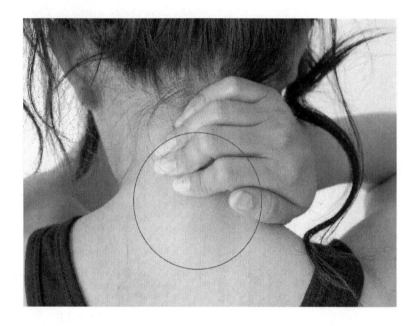

CAN DISMAL POSTURE POINT US TOWARDS A DISEASED STATE?

Think back to the previous chapters when the relevance of structure interfering with nerve function was discussed. Now that you have a better understanding of the nature of connective tissue, this should come as no surprise. We can appreciate that the body is a self-healing and self-regulating system. The big question now is whether bad posture can affect the biophoton emission of your body. The fact that the fascia sheaths become tacky and ropey is just the body's way of dealing with stress and stabilizing your posture. The only problem here is that, past a point in time, adhesions in one place may create strain or compensation in another. For example, a stressed liver may form restrictive shoulder or knee patterns. As you can see, our spine, nervous system and connective tissues play a vital part in our posture and our overall health; the more it functions properly, the more stable our health potential is.

> *"Better than 90 percent of the energy output of the brain is used in relating to the physical body in its gravitational field. The more mechanically distorted a person is, the less energy available for thinking, metabolism and healing."*
> —*Dr. Roger Sperry, Nobel Laureate*

There is much biophotonic research done worldwide on both improving cellular communication and breaking bad communication patterns. In over thirty years of healthcare, Lawrence has come to the conclusion that the cells lose energy (cellular vibration) too-much or too-little cell-to-cell communication may be one of the major contributors (cellular communication) in the chronic disease process.

Cellular vibration: If your cellular vibrations are optimal, you are much healthier because you are functioning at ideal level – your body is firing on all cylinders. For example, imagine that you have a pickup truck and you're driving slowly down a 'bad' neighborhood street. Chances are, you may get some unwanted passengers (germs, cancer, etc.). Alternatively, if you are zipping down that same street with your truck, nobody can jump on.

Cellular communication: Cells talk to each other by using light. The coherent emission of biophotons is connected to information transfer processes in the cells, and has been linked to the function of DNA and to gene regulation.

By using light as a medium to energize cells and improve cellular communication, the potential could be limitless. In terms of healing the implications are colossal. We now know, for example, that quanta of light can initiate, or arrest, cascade-like reactions in the cells, and that genetic cellular damage can be virtually repaired, within hours, by faint beams of light. Recollect in the beginning of this chapter where new-borns with jaundice were treated with blue lights. The frequency of the blue lights resonate with frequency of the liver cells to promote healing.

It is unfortunate that our 'mainstream medicine' hasn't advanced this area in terms of treatment. Paradoxically, doctors accept, believe and trust technologies such as MRI, PET scans, CAT scan, X-ray, ECG, EKG, diagnostic ultrasound, etc. Aren't these diagnostic procedures generally using the same biophotonic principles (electromagnetic field)?

Unfortunately, biophotonics, in terms of application, is often side-stepped and is usually mistakenly labelled as 'alternative' or energy medicine. Alternative energy practitioners generally profess to be 'clearing', 'moving', 'astral changing', and 'purifying' energy fields of the body. But what does that mean and are these based on anything? Although people many people may find benefit from energy work, these techniques are mostly subjective and are usually particularly difficult to quantify.

On one hand we have the medical societies professing not to use or believe in energy but in actual fact use it all day long as 'scientific' diagnostic tools, and on the other hand we have these others pontificating 'unscientific' energy treatments. Hmmm, where's the logic here? It doesn't matter if the practitioner believes in the energy or not. He or she is probably using it in some form all day without even understanding it nor connecting the dots about it. A further inconsistency here is that the medic's diagnosis is based on the electromagnetic field but the treatment is generally administered in the form of a biochemical substance. There is plenty of room here for brave intelligent students to blaze a new trail in this field for the purposes of treatment and application.

5

Sedentary Society – Our Changing Lifestyle and Its Impact on Posture

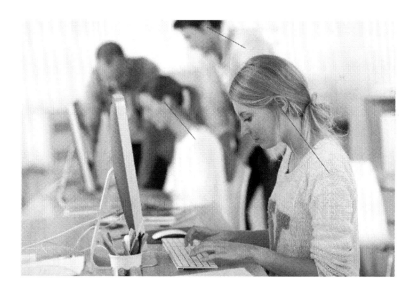

In recent years, research on sedentary routines has increased to out-of-control levels and there is cascading evidence that a multitude of serious health risks are connected to sedentary lifestyles. Recent studies warn that sedentary lifestyles are likely to be causing as many deaths as smoking.

Unfortunately, most adults spend a large portion of each day in a seated position as well. It's hard to avoid these days, as computer work predominates, and most also spend many precious hours each week commuting to and from work, constantly checking their phones. A 2006 study found that 32% of the population spends more than 10 hours a day seated. Half do not leave their desks, even to have lunch. Two thirds of people also sit down at home when they get home from work.*

* The Way You Sit Will Never Be the Same! Alterations of Lumbosacral Curvature and Intervertebral Disc Morphology in Normal Subjects in Variable Sitting Positions Using Whole-body Positional MRI, Waseem Bashir MBChB, Tetsuya Torio MD, Francis Smith MD, Keisuke Takahashi, Malcolm Pope PhD; 2006

Sitting actually increases the pressure on the lower vertebrae by three times or more as compared to standing or lying down. Our bodies normally have natural curve, but when we are using laptops, tablets, and phones we tend to be more forward in our posture. Our shoulders get rounded. When this becomes a habit, the vertebrae can get out of alignment leading to subluxation (misalignments of the bones leading to nerve interference). Our joints begin to break down and with enough time and stress leads to bone spurs and fusions. This breakdown causes interference in the way the nervous and collagen systems communicates, thus producing pain and discomfort, illness, disease, and loss of function.

The 'actively sedentary' is a new normal of individuals who are fit for one hour but sitting around the rest of the day. However, as the studies have shown, you simply cannot counterbalance sitting all day with exercise.

Complacent Posture Adaption Over Time

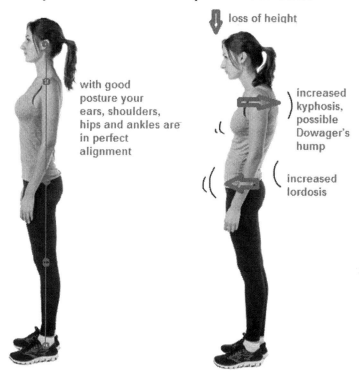

loss of height

with good posture your ears, shoulders, hips and ankles are in perfect alignment

increased kyphosis, possible Dowager's hump

increased lordosis

FOR THOSE SITTING ABOVE 8 – 10 HOURS PER DAY, THE FOLLOWING ARE THE TOP 10 HEALTH RISKS:

1. Cardiovascular Health

* Proper KI, Singh AS, van Mechelen W, et al. Sedentary behaviors and health outcomes among adults: a systematic review of prospective studies. American journal of preventive medicine 2011;40(2):174-82.

2. Cancer

* Biswas A, Oh PI, Faulkner GE, et al. Sedentary time and its association with risk for disease incidence, mortality, and hospitalization in adults: a systematic review and meta-analysis. Annals of internal medicine 2015;162(2):123-32.

3. Diabetes (Type 2)

* De Rezende, L. F. M., Rodrigues Lopes, M., Rey-López, J. P., Matsudo, V. K. R., & Luiz, O. do C. (2014). Sedentary behavior and health outcomes: An overview of systematic reviews. PLoS ONE, 9, doi:10.1371/journal.pone.0105620.

4. Weight Gain

* Smith L, Thomas EL, Bell JD, et al. The association between objectively measured sitting and standing with body composition: a pilot study using MRI. BMJ open 2014;4(6):e005476.

5. Metabolic Syndrome

* Greer, A.E., Sui, X., Maslow, A.L., Greer, B.K. & Blair, S.N. (2015). The effects of sedentary behavior on metabolic syndrome independent of physical activity and cardiorespiratory fitness. J Phys Act Health, 12, 68-73, doi: 10.1123/jpah.2013-0186.

6. Mental Health

* Hamer M, Coombs N, Stamatakis E. Associations between objectively assessed and self-reported sedentary time with mental health in adults: an analysis of data from the Health Survey for England. BMJ open 2014;4(3):e004580.

7. Back/Neck Pain

* Roffey DM, Wai EK, Bishop P, et al. Causal assessment of occupational standing or walking and low back pain: results of a systematic review. The spine journal : official journal of the North American Spine Society 2010;10(3):262-72.

8. Muscle Degeneration

* Hamer M, Stamatakis E. Screen-based sedentary behavior, physical activity, and muscle strength in the English longitudinal study of ageing. PloS one 2013;8(6):e66222.

9. Osteoporosis

* Chastin SFM, Mandrichenko O, Helbostadt JL, et al. Associations between objectively-measured sedentary behaviour and physical activity with bone mineral density in adults and older adults, the NHANES study. Bone 2014;64:254-62.

10. Mortality

* Proper KI, Singh AS, van Mechelen W, et al. Sedentary behaviors and health outcomes among adults: a systematic review of prospective studies. American journal of preventive medicine 2011;40(2):174-82.

According to Dr. James Levine, 'For every hour that you sit, your life expectancy decreases by two hours.* By comparison, every cigarette smoked reduces life expectancy by eleven minutes.' This means that sitting is far more dangerous than smoking! Adults are also susceptible to exacerbations that can further impact their posture, such as stress and low energy. For many adults, the stress of the world weighs heavily on them, and the burden of that weight is often reflected in their posture.

*Get Up!: Why Your Chair is Killing You and What You Can Do About It by James A. Levine

Another study from the American Journal of Pain Management*, poor posture and back problems can impact every physiological function from breathing to hormone production. It has been shown that posture can influence mood, blood pressure, pulse, lung capacity or whether you have a headache or not. The functions most profoundly influenced by posture are respiration, oxygenation and sympathetic nervous system function. It also appears that homeostasis and autonomic regulation are inextricably linked to posture. The corollary of these interpretations is that many common ailments, including pain, may be moderated or even eliminated by enhanced posture.

*Lennon et al. (1994). Posture and Respiratory Modulation of Autonomic Function, Pain, and Health. American Journal of Pain Management. 4 (36-39).

It is the lack of a proper movement and complacent body positions, and not lack of exercise, which are predominant contributors to poor posture in adults. While most teens are able to maintain their shape without being active, adults have a more difficult time maintaining muscle mass, which is a prerequisite for proper spine alignment. As we age, movement becomes increasingly important in our efforts to prevent body decompensation. When the body stops moving for prolonged periods of time, it's like telling your body it's time to stop working and prepare for breakdown.

LET'S EXAMINE WHAT GOES ON
INTERNALLY WITH A SEDENTARY BODY:

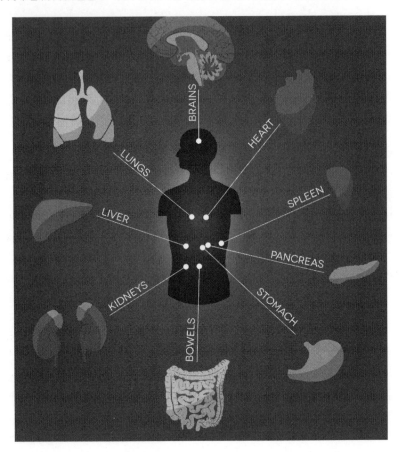

- **Strained Neck and Shoulders**: Statistically, everyone holds their neck and head forward while working with gadgets (media). This ultimately leads to strains in your neck, which can lead to neck degeneration.
- **Cartilage:** Sitting puts more pressure on the joints and discs of the spine instead of placing stress on the foundational muscles. The strain is exacerbated if you sit hunched over in front of your computer.
- **Spinal Discs**: The discs in your back are meant to expand and contract as you move. This allows nutrients and oxygen to be absorbed through imbibition. Sitting improperly compresses the discs, which can lead to breakdown and herniation.

- **Muscles**: Movement involves the engagement of foundational muscles. These muscles disengage when you sit, ultimately leading to atrophy.
- **Pelvis:** Your pelvis also degenerates from persistent sitting. The muscles tighten and the range of motion diminishes due to a perpetual flexion of the hips. Gluteal muscle atrophy can subsequently limit your ability to run or jump.
- **Bones**: Weight-bearing activities lead to stronger, denser bones. Lack of activity may cause weak bones and, ultimately, osteoporosis.
- **Pancreas:** Your body's ability to respond to insulin is affected by just one day of excess sitting, which leads your pancreas to producing increased amounts of insulin.
- **Heart**: When you sit, the blood flow diminishes and muscles don't burn as much fat, which makes it easier for fatty acids to obstruct your heart.
- **Colon:** Excess sitting may increase your risk of colon, breast and endometrial cancers. It also increases the risk of colon cancer by 30% and of uterine cancer by 66%.*
- **Lungs:** Prolonged sitting increases the chances of lung cancer by 54%.*
- **Digestion:** Sitting down after you've eaten causes your abdominal contents to compress, slowing down digestion and ultimately leading to digestive disorders.*
- **Brain:** Your brain function brakes when your body sits for too long. Your brain will get a lesser amount of fresh blood and oxygen, which are needed to activate the release of brain- and mood-enhancing chemicals.
- **Sensory:** Most of this pain can be traced directly to our proclivity to live sedentary lifestyles. An important principle to internalize is that pain is usually an indicator that something is wrong. We know that even a rigorous exercise regimen is not sufficient to compensate for the damage being caused by prolonged sitting. * Findings presented at the 2015 Inaugural Active Working Summit themindunleashed.com/2015/04/this-is-what-sitting-for-too-long-can-do-to-your-body.html

6

Children

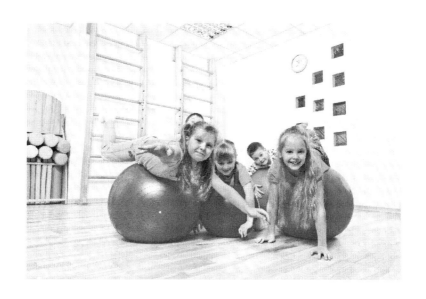

The body is as young as the spine is supple.'
—Indian Proverb

One generation ago, children used to play outside all day, riding bikes, playing sports, climbing trees and neighborhood games that didn't require planning or adult supervision. Children of the past spent most of their time outdoors and their sensory world was elementary and modest. The family time was often spent at the dinner table, where everyone sat together and actually spoke to one another about their day. Children had chores and other expectations that had to be met. Life was relatively simple.

*the author prefers to use the term 'children' and not 'kids'. Words are powerful and, if we look etymologically at what the word 'kids' means...

Today's generation is different. Technology's influence on the 'modern' family is rocking its core, thus creating a fragmentation of the very fundamental values that have been the bedrock of society for many generations. People are frantically trying to manage (for the sake of making things faster and more efficient) work, school, 'playdates', adult supervised activities for their children, and technology. The flaming fireplace has been replaced by the flickering media screen. And who needs a home cooked meal that takes hours to prepare when you can simply go to a drive-through or take-away? Children no longer need to go outside to see nature. They can sit on the couch and experience their world through the lens of smart devices, i-devices, video games and other media gizmos.

This dramatic change in lifestyle is related to our youth's overreliance on technology, which has made the lives of our children increasingly sedentary. In fact, a recent study of 12,000 parents in 10 countries suggest that inmates spend more time outdoors than children.* They are also increasingly dependent on technology such as phones, computers, video games and television, which ultimately leads to the development of poor posture. Lastly, our children's schoolbags seem to getting larger and heavier.

*Research was conducted by Edelman Berland, an independent market research firm. Fieldwork was conducted in February and March 2016 in US, Brazil, UK, Turkey, Portugal, South Africa, Vietnam, China, Indonesia, and India.

Another appalling study* showed that elementary aged children use on average 7.5 hours per day of entertainment technology, 75 percent of these children have TV's in their bedrooms, and 50 percent of North

American homes have the TV on all day! Our children cannot contrast a world without media gadgets and gizmos, but parents should. Therefore the only possible solution begins with changing these patterns at home.

*Kaiser Family Foundation Study; JANUARY 2010, GENERATION M2, Media in the lives of 8- to 18-Year-Olds; Victoria J. Rideout, M.A, Ulla G. Foehr, Ph.D

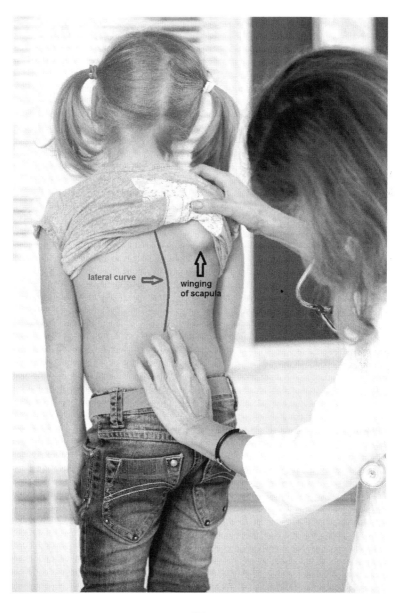

"As the twig is bent, so is the tree,"
—B.J. Palmer

The author now sees children in his practice who present with conditions that were previously only seen in adults. The structural collapse of the skeleton may play a contributing role in a myriad of aches, pains and unexplained health problems. The skeleton is the framework of support for all the body's systems, including nervous, circulatory, respiratory, and digestive system functions. The question is, how can we correct these problems and make sure that children grow up to have good posture?

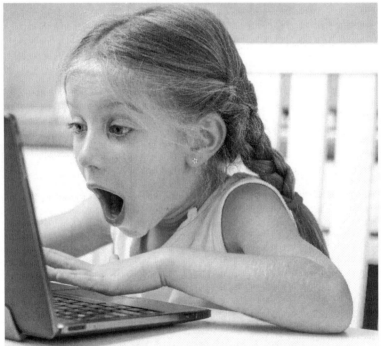

change has to begin at home

SOME SUGGESTIONS FOR CHILDREN:

Perhaps you recall your parents telling you to sit up straight and now you find yourself telling your children the same thing. 'Straighten up!' or 'Stop slouching' still echo through the halls of many households. Eventually, children will grow into adults, and these poor movement patterns will have become deeply ingrained. How can we turn this around?

Let's start by breaking this down into typical childhood activities and how we and optimize their environment. **Proper posture habits should be on par with brushing your teeth, eating good food, and a good night's sleep**. Awareness of this potential problem is a good place to start.

Home: At home we can educate children of proper posture hygiene by using seat wedges designed especially for children; ergonomic balls instead of couches; movement every 15 minutes; Of course, encouraging children to go outside playing is always the best option. Remember, (logic again) your children will mirror your behavior so you turn your phone off too and get moving.

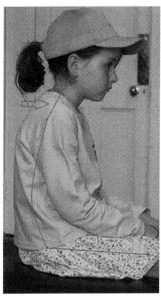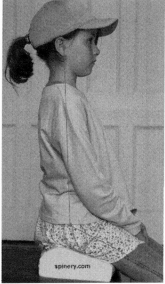

Technological Device Use: Living in the contemporary digital age certainly has it's benefits. It makes you wonder, how did we ever live without the endless amounts of information at our fingertips? However, with all the benefits we gain from modern-day technology, we are witnessing unprecedented and serious risks of perpetual health compli-cations, such as 'text neck'. Unfortunately, texting is now part of our culture and it appears that it is here to stay. The best recommendation is simply awareness of the problem. If you or your child needs to use a media device, try to keep it up at eye level **and put time limits on these devices**.

Sitting: Many experts propose a solution that children can simply counter the degenerative effects of disproportionate sitting by standing. This may be true to a certain extent, but there are also some potential downsides to standing in the same position for long periods of time. If you stand in an inactive posture for a prolonged period, you may overload your spine, which can cause back pain. Ideally, you should strive for a balance between sitting, standing and moving. One of the best ways to do this is to monitor their sitting, standing and moving times.

School: Lawrence recommends for teachers to introduce this by using an egg timer so that they are reminded to move every 15 minutes. Even if the child just stands and sits, this may be enough to reboot. The alternation of sitting, standing and moving is not a panacea, but every-thing counts when it comes to your health.

Backpacks: Backpacks are getting bigger and heavier and not in propor-tion to the size of children. You can recognize when a child's backpack is too heavy if he or she has to lean their head forward while carrying it in order to sustain balance. Remember, for every inch of forward head position compared to the neutral position, the weight of the head increases by 10 pounds on the spine.* This forward head position has been linked to many modern day health problems.

* Kapandji, Physiology of Joints, Vol. 3

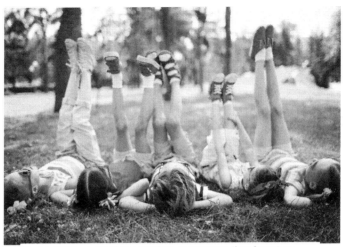
Wouldn't it be great if our children spent more time in nature using their imaginations and creativity rather than being plugged into a device?

Another study* concludes that backpack loads are accountable for a substantial amount of back pain in children. The same study says that a full third of children aged 11 to 14 report back pain. Other studies also indicate that a backpack should be no more than 10 percent of your child's entire body weight. For children under 10 years of age, the backpack's weight should be closer to five percent of your child's body weight. Even though these researchers have come to these conclusions, do you really think that a child can handle 10 percent of their body weight? For example, according to this study, it would be sufficient for a ten-year-old weighing 80 pounds to carry the equivalent of a 8 pound sack of potatoes on his or her back. Despite the findings in this study, can we logically assume that this individual will develop a poor posture pattern over time?

* Spine; 2010 Jan 1;35(1):83-8.

Poor posture with backpacks can not only cause chronic back pain, but one may begin to unconsciously assume these dysfunctional body patterns even when they're not carrying a backpack. When this occurs, the child is no longer 'consciously' adapting to his or her environment, and their body begins to complacently adapt to these dysfunctional structural patterns. The rest is predictable. It typically starts with a pain somewhere, be it the neck, shoulder, lower back and so forth, and the pain eventually leads to a chronic condition.

We all clearly see this as a problem. Schools are increasing standards and raising the level of homework assignments, which may mean more books to take home. However, do they have to bring everything home every night? Additionally, rather than heave the entire load around all day, perhaps most books can be left in the child's locker, provided there is enough time between classes. Homework can be assigned per subject per night.

Some schools have combatted the issue of excessive load by distributing extra copies of textbooks, so that children don't have to carry as many books between school and home. School districts are increasingly beginning to issue texts on thumb drives or in digital format. However, encouraging the use of personal computers and tablets among children creates a whole new set of problems.

The author has given training on good posture to local schools in his community. Education should be delivered with an understanding of the human body, biomechanics and how postural changes can occur and be managed. Lawrence worked directly with one small school in Ireland, where the author and a colleague dedicated an entire year of their lives to educate students on good posture and how to re-learn primal movement patterns.

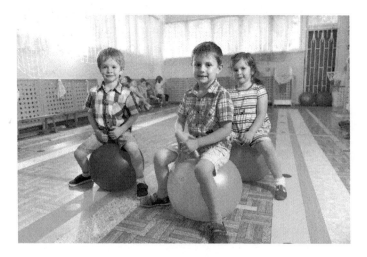

Throughout that year, students and faculty were presented with ways to incorporate proper posture into their existing systems and curriculum. This school even went so far as to remove all of the chairs from the premises and replace them with ergonomic balls. Though there was some resistance to this dramatic change (from both teachers and students), eventually everyone settled, and the results of this seemingly small change were incredible. Students became more alert and attentive and demonstrated an increased capacity to absorb information. The number of children who normally had difficulty concentrating was greatly reduced, and the students' increased efficiency in the classroom afforded them more opportunities to engage in fun and exciting activities outside of it.

The author is most excited about the research that he has conducted with regard to backpacks. He and his staff used to monitor the effects of backpacks (and prolonged sitting) in his office. The children and adults in his research were scanned before and after carrying a backpack, and after the transition from seated to standing. The scan measured the electrical activity of the muscles in and around the spine. The author found that, if the placement of the schoolbag deviated at a certain angle, the stress was then transferred from the spine to the foundation muscles (hips). Additionally, when the seat angle was changed to a certain degree, again, the stress went off the spine to the foundation muscles. From these studies, the author engineered a solution that tackles both of these issues at once.

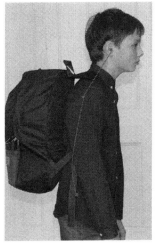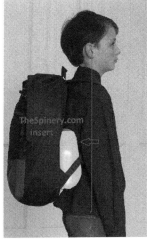

The Spinery's Foundation® transfers the stress off of the spine while carrying a bag and/or when seated. By taking the stress off of the spine and distributing it to the core muscles, the back is protected and proper posture is maintained.

"The beginning of the disease process starts with postural distortions."
—*Dr. Hans Seyle, Nobel Laureate*

Children's Car Seats – Long before children start carrying backpacks or gazing at media apparatuses, they're forced into car seats and strollers that can play a major role in the development of postural problems. If we examine how babies teach themselves how to sit up, we notice that they attempt to put their weight on the part of the pelvis that puts the sacrum at the proper angle to support the spine. This position allows the spine to align itself along the vertical axis of gravity such that it can sustain a heavy head balanced on top. Once a child discovers this position, sitting upright is effortless and proper. However, car seats and strollers force the child's pelvis into a reverse tilted position (opposite of what is optimal). This disturbs the angle of the pelvis in relation to the spine, causing the spine to slouch (lordotic curve).

A reverse tilting pelvis causes the muscles in the front of the body to shorten, thus creating habits that are perpetually reinforced until they become the new default position that governs how those muscles will function. As the child develops, this shortening in the front of the body becomes so ingrained in a child's musculature that it not only defines how the child moves currently, but also how he or she will age in the future. Again, only advice here is awareness of the problem and try to reduce exposure.

CHAPTER

7

Analyze Yourself

LET'S START BY EVALUATING YOUR ALIGNMENT:

Statistically, nobody pays attention to their postural changes or deviations. To move forward you simply must take an objective view of yourself so that *you* can fix *you*. So, put on your workout gear and ask a friend to take two full-body photos, one from the front and one from the side. Keep your muscles relaxed, but stand as tall as you can, with your feet hip-width apart and with your hands hanging normally at your sides. Try to stand normally and don't assume 'good posture' or the 'military stance.' Now compare your photos with the illustrations below to analyze your posture problems. Note body type and then the following checkpoints relative to a lateral plumb line falling just anterior (front) to the external malleolus (ankle) and an anterior (front) or posterior (back) vertical line between the heels. Later, we will follow this with repair plans.

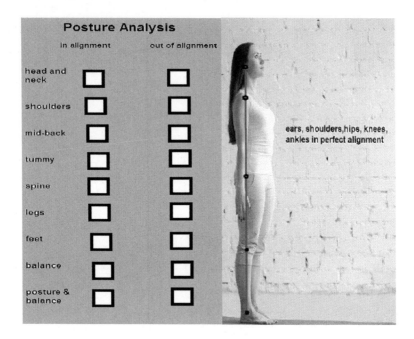

Head and Neck: Your ear should be directly over the middle of your shoulder – if your ear is not directly over, but in front of your shoulder, you have forward head posture. For every inch your head posture goes forward, your head becomes 10 pounds 'heavier' on the muscles and bones of the neck. From the rear, note the position of your head. If the head is tilted to the right, the chin will tilt to the left and vice versa. Note the symmetry of the neck muscles. Now look at the bottom of the ears – if one is higher than the other often indicates a head tilt and a sign of possible neck misalignment.

Shoulders: Look at the shoulders; they should be level, and if they are not, this is a sign of a mid-back misalignment. From the side, note the rotation or tilting of the lower angles of the shoulder blade (scapulae). From the rear, observe the comparative height of the scapulae, comparing one to the other. Check for winged shoulder blade or for scapulae failing to lie smoothly on your back. The mid-back (thoracic spine) is always curved toward the side on which the scapula is more prominent and flaring. If the shoulder is high on the right and the scapula flares on the right, the entire neck and mid-back is curved toward the right. If the shoulder is high on the right, yet the right shoulder blade flares, the neck is typically curved to the left and the mid-back is curved to the left.

Mid-back: From the front, observe any signs of hollow chest, sternal or rib depression, or pathologic signs, such as barrel chest or pigeon chest. From the rear, note the contours of the neck and shoulder muscles for customary development or for atypical tightness or tenderness. Note the angles of the ribs. A difference in the height of the shoulder blades and the hip (iliac) crests usually indicates a curvature of the spine (scoliosis). Lateral positions of the spinous processes and anterior or posterior positions of the transverse processes together with an elevation of the angles of the ribs indicate a rotation of the spinal bones (vertebra).

Tummy: From the side, check the degree of stomach muscle relaxation. Keep in mind that children normally have a prominent tummy and adult women have a deposit of superficial fat lying diagonally below the belly button.

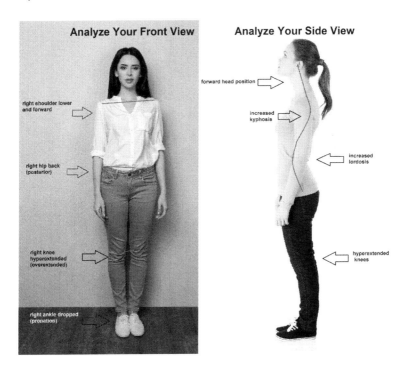

Spine: Check the curvatures of the spine from a side view. Look for accentuated curves (lordotic or kyphotic). Note the degree of the pelvis (sacral tilt and lumbosacral angle). From the rear, compare the line of the spinal bones. Evaluate any side spinal curves (scoliosis).

Legs: From the side, note the degree of the alignment of the knee. Note if your knees are locking or pushing backwards (hyperextension) – this can often cause damaged ligaments, cartilage and other stabilizing structures in the knee. From the front, check for any degree of the knees pointing in or out.

Feet: Notice the alignment. Is one foot slightly behind the other or flaring out? Are your arches dropping? By the way, there are many causes of flattened arches, but one of the key culprits is that the gluteal muscles are usually extremely weak on the flat foot side. Therefore, by strengthening the gluteal muscles, the legs should eventually return to a proper alignment from the hips down and, therefore, slowly raises the arches back to correct levels.

Now Let's Check your Balance:

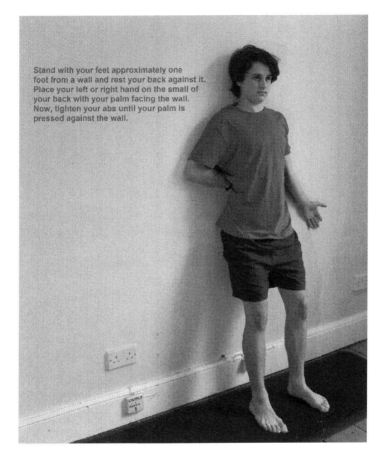

Stand with your feet approximately one foot from a wall and rest your back against it. Place your left or right hand on the small of your back with your palm facing the wall. Now, tighten your abs until your palm is pressed against the wall.

Place your hands on top of your hips. If one hip is higher than the other, this could be a sign of misalignment of your lower back or hip. Note the comparative height of your hips. Check the comparative height and depth of the sacral dimples and the bilateral buttock height. If chronic sciatica is on the high hip (iliac crest side), degenerative disc weakening should be suspected. If it occurs on the side of the hip (low iliac crest), one must consider the possibility of a sacroiliac slip and/ or mechanical alignment as being the causative factor.

Standing with your feet square and toes forward, place a straightedge or ruler flat on the inside of your foot so that it is straight up and touching the bony protrusion on the inside of your ankle. If in alignment, this straight edge should also be touching the fleshy part of the top of your arch as it goes straight down from the bony protrusion on the inside of your ankle. The bigger the space is between the ruler or straightedge and the skin of your arch, the flatter your foot is.

Stand with your feet approximately one foot from a wall and rest your back against it. Place your left or right hand on the small of your back, palm facing the wall. Then, tighten your abs until your palm is pressed against the wall. In this position, your body should have four points of contact with the wall: your tailbone, palm, upper back and head. If you have to tilt your head back to reach the wall, you may have a problem. The most likely scenario is that the abs and chest muscles have shortened, while your posterior chain muscles and spine have weakened. Sitting (incorrectly) for extended periods of time leads to this imbalance.

LASTLY, EXAMINE YOUR POSTURE AND BALANCE:

Your awareness of where you think you are in space and the true reality of where you actually are:

Stand up straight and lift your left knee so your foot comes off the ground. Slowly count to 20 and stop the first time you (1) have to put your foot down, (2) move your arms, (**if you find yourself throwing your arms out or twisting about, chances are that you're showing signs of weak balance**), (3) start to lean to one side.

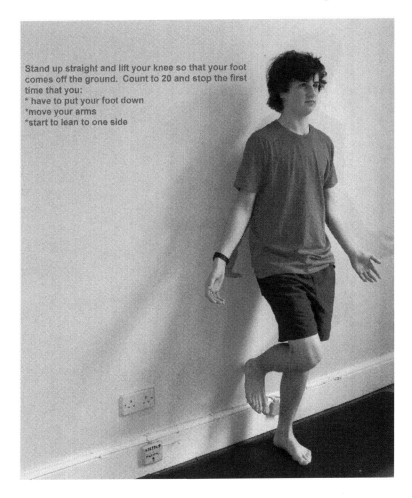

Stand up straight and lift your knee so that your foot comes off the ground. Count to 20 and stop the first time that you:
* have to put your foot down
*move your arms
*start to lean to one side

Repeat this test on both sides. How long can you balance on your right or left leg?

Now, lift one leg as you balance on the other. You should be able to balance on each leg for at least thirty seconds. If you cannot, your body may not be functioning as well as it should.

CHAPTER

8

Solutions – Active Conscious Engagement (ACE)

The good news is that most of you have the capacity to get yourself out of chronic pain and attain a more vibrant and youthful body than you ever imagined possible. However, it will require that you relearn appropriate movement patterns and discard deeply entrenched poor posture habits.

Getting structurally sound doesn't need to be an ostentatious or complex task. It's really quite simple. It only relies on only you, your movements, and your breathing. Through a sequence of postures, seated positions, and movements, the following techniques will adapt you to take the weight of your body away from your discs and joints and direct it to your foundational muscles. In other words, your body will now be trading a tree trunk for a toothpick. As you do these techniques, you will begin to notice your alignment. Also, try to feel all of your core muscles engaging. This will also engage your brain so that by doing these primal movements and postures, your muscles will become actively engaged all the time (i.e. while sitting, brushing your teeth, or even walking the dog).

Most of us would agree that the majority of people live in their heads. Be it driving your children to school, at work, squeezing in grocery shopping, never mind the elephant in the room (media). For example, look around you right now and observe how many people are fixated on a media screen of some sort. This has got to be the biggest reason why our bodies are losing consciousness. The only time that we may actually try to connect with the body is the few hours a week when we may go to a gym, exercise class, guru, etc.

What if we turned all of this around? What if you used your imagination to make every movement a conscious and active engagement? For example, if you are seated properly, you should feel your stomach muscles engaged (as well as every foundation muscle). Eventually, you should no longer need to be doing any of the techniques, because, as the gurus say, 'you are.' If you're old enough to remember the film 'The Karate Kid,' there was this young boy who was put through a series of exercises, but he didn't know why. Ultimately, this character found out that, if you pursue mastership, there is nothing left to learn. By adopting this philosophy, you will logically move to higher ground and these patterns will become proper and primal.

Being *conscious* of your body is the most important step to change. An active conscious engaged (ACE) posture is when you know and can feel the specific place for your body to be bio-mechanically strong. The key is strengthening your posture with deliberate movements. We have a lot of options for exercises with ACE that can correct our postural deviation. However, it may be recommended that you seek professional advice as to which specific exercise is appropriate for a particular case. Suffering from an injury due to inappropriate exercise is the last thing that you'd want to happen. Thus, it is important to follow the recommendation of your therapist and perform each exercise religiously. Remember, posture cannot be corrected overnight. Have patience. After all, once you see the results of your hard work, it will all be worth it. Try to invent your own active conscious engagement exercises. Everyone's body is unique. Ultimately, you should become the expert of your own body.

Consciously engaged posture is quite literally how you balance your mind and body. There are countless arrangements of possible joint configurations that result in a body balancing itself. But relax, no one has 'perfect' posture. The objective for robust posture is to strive towards the best possible biomechanical orientation of the body where all the muscles and joints are ideally aligned to function as well as possible while coherently stressing the foundation muscles and not the joints or discs. In other words, the power of your posture is how well you know and control where your body is in space.

With perfect posture, your head, shoulders, hips, knees, and ankles are all aligned. When you're standing, and walking, and moving, no matter how you're using your body, it's the foundational muscles engagement and coupling up and down the kinetic chain that minimizes injury and maximizes performance.

Here's the contradiction though....the point of doing exercises is that eventually you won't need to do them anymore. With that in mind, when re-learning primal movement patterns, it is best to break things down to their essence and engage your mind until proper movement becomes subconscious. The goal is to actively engage your foundation muscles while walking, sitting, brushing your teeth, etc

Use the following exercises that Lawrence has given as a pointer or guide. Also use your creative skills and adapt these exercises to suit your needs. These exercises are not meant to focus on individual muscles. They are designed to synchronously engage the anterior (front) and posterior (back) muscles chains collectively. It is best to do this in front of a mirror to check your alignment. In all of these exercises, we want to stretch and strengthen the muscles simultaneously by activating the antagonist chain of muscles and stretching the agonist chain of muscles. In other words, stretch and strengthen your structure in proper alignment.

THE PRIMAL PATTERNING:

Let's start with a primal movement pattern which can be done through-out the day. The goal here is to incorporate this movement pattern in to how you stand, walk, sit and everything else. Remember, mastery comes by repetition. The more that you move in these primal movement patterns, the more you will become actively and consciously engaged in all of your daily activities.

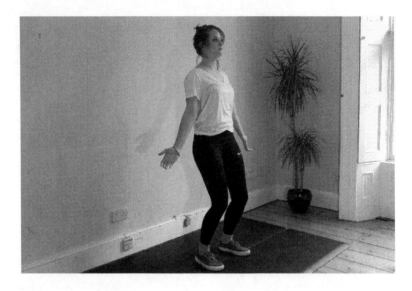

Begin by placing your feet shoulder-width apart and slightly bend your knees, with your weight on your heels, arms off to the side with externally rotated hands. Take a few deep breaths as you hold this position. Try to assume this posture as much as you can throughout your day. Also, when you stand, always keep your knees slightly flexed, just enough to feel your muscles engage. Always practice doing this and you will begin to transfer all of the stress from your spine (backbone) unto your muscles. Just doing this alone will drive you into a conscious state of mind.

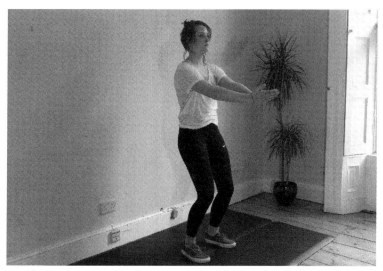

From that same position, bring your hands together, maintaining your weight on your heels. Your ears should be even with your shoulders, hips and ankles. Your palms facing up. Take a deep breath. Close your eyes – can you feel all of your muscles engaging?

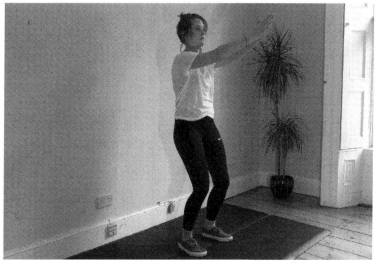

Now, in that same position, with your weight balanced on your heels, bring your arms up and lift up (extend) your rib cage as well (be careful not to extend or flex the spine, keep it vertical), and hold this position for 10 seconds while taking deep breaths.

Active Conscious Engaged Sitting:

Now let's look at you sit. Imagine taking a wooden ruler and bending it. When you bend the ruler, you create stress along the length of the ruler. The stress on the ruler is greatest at the exact point of the bend. If you continue to bend the ruler, it will eventually break. Sitting with poor posture stresses the spine in a similar way. When you sit, the spine is slumped forward and this places enormous stress on the discs and joints, which is the source of most back pain.

Postural deviations lead to improper joint wear, arthritis, muscle imbalances, disc degeneration, and often to metabolic disease. Not to mention how they physically affect the way you present yourself and the degree of confidence your body displays. Therefore, postural correction should be the primary focus in any activity. Whenever you feel any tension, fatigue, discomfort or even pain, the first thing you should always do is check in on your posture. Practice your sitting and move-ment posture as if your quality of life depends on it – because it certainly does! So, notice the way you are sitting. Is the back curved, shoulders slumped, maybe even legs crossed?

Good Sitting Technique:

You will do less harm by sitting upright on the front edge of your chair with your knees slightly below the hips. Backrests tend to promote undue round-ing of the spine and tend to push people into a forward-head-translation. The further forward your head goes, the shorter your hip flexors will remain, and that just leads to all sorts of mechanical problems.

When sitting for a while, try to keep your chest bone (sternum) in front of your chin. As soon as the head starts to fall forward, your discs enter the compression/degeneration zone. Consider lengthening the distance between the rib cage and the pelvis when you stand. This will elongate your hip flexors.

Some research recommends standing up for two minutes every 20 minutes you spend sitting down and standing up during commercials when watching TV. The 'jury is still out' on the long-term effects of sitting – standing but it does seem that the less time spent sitting, the better off you will be.

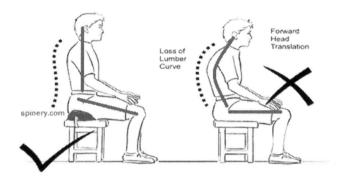

Let's look at some research summaries:

A 1999 study was completed to develop a new sitting spinal model and an optimal driver's seat by using review of the literature of seated positions of the head, spine, pelvis, and lower extremities. The conclusion was that the low back forward curvature (lumbar lordosis) is affected by the trunk-thigh angle and the knee angle. The subjects in seats with backrest inclinations of **110 to 130 degrees**, with concomitant lumbar support, **have the lowest disc pressures and lowest electromyography recordings from spinal muscles.**[*]Journal of Manipulative and Physiological Therapeutics 22(9):594-609 November 1999

Another study by Scottish and Canadian researchers found that sitting up straight places an unnecessary strain on your back, due to the strain put on the spine and its associated ligaments over time, thus causing pain, deformity and chronic illness. The conclusion of this study found that disc movement was found to be most pronounced with a 90-degree upright sitting posture. It was least pronounced with the 135-degree posture, suggesting less strain is placed on the spinal disks and associated muscles and tendons in a more relaxed sitting position.[*] The Way You Sit Will Never Be the Same! Alterations of Lumbosacral Curvature and Intervertebral Disc Morphology in Normal Subjects in Variable Sitting Positions Using Whole-body Positional MRI Waseem Bashir MBChB, Tetsuya Torio MD, Francis Smith MD, Keisuke Takahashi, Malcolm Pope PhD; 2006

If you think about it, these studies make sense. The human body is a biological entity which is non-linear. The notion of a chair with ninety-degree angles is incongruous with how we are designed.

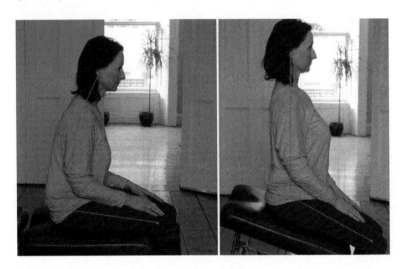

A seated position with hips and back in flexion. This is a complacent position, in which spinal muscles are complacently engaged, and the foundation muscles are disengaged.

A seated position in which the ears, shoulders and hips align with the knees below the hips, thus creating an 'active' posture in which the foundation muscles are engaged **(ACE).** Try this yourself. Arrange you seat in which your knees are below your hips. Can you feel that you are now using your muscles and not your spine to sit? Do you feel what muscles you are now using? Close your eyes and notice your hands and feet. Sitting in this position requires no volition on your part to sit proper. Now all of your foundation muscles are engaged and sitting like this is actually beneficial to the body. You are actively and consciously engaged.

Some people want to know what chair they should buy to keep the hips above the knees. The author has searched high and low to find the perfect chair without much success. Trouble is that it seems that chair manufacturers start with the idea for a chair and not the human frame. The chair in the picture below was designed by the author (www.thespinery.com). This chair was designed with the human frame and human mechanics in mind in order to actively engage foundation muscles while seated.

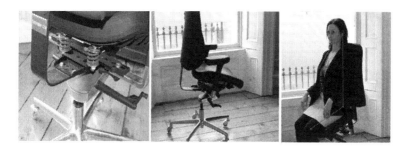

Alternatively, if you're not that ambitious, perhaps sit on a seat wedge. If you are going to purchase a seat wedge, try to find the orthopedic insert with high density foam in the range of 5.0 to 5.5 lb/ft3. Don't be fooled by the descriptions 'orthopedic' or 'doctor recommended', you be the ultimate arbiter. The wedge should be firm for support and have some molding properties to increase surface area. The author has yet to find a seat wedge available that meets his criteria in terms of both appropriate foam density and correct angle. Again, you might need to make your own. In the following picture is the seat wedge that Lawrence makes fusing high density and gel foams for his patients to actively engage their foundation muscles while seated:

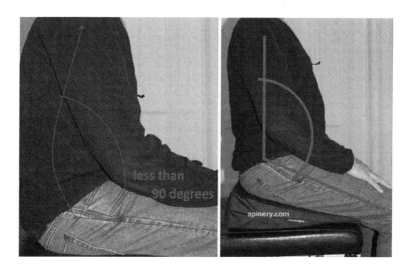

ACTIVE CONSCIOUS ENGAGED STANDING:

Generally good standing posture (from a side view) is a straight line from middle of the ear to your ankle. The frontal view should demonstrate a straight spine and level hips, shoulders and head.

For achieving a good standing posture, here's an excellent exercise and stretch: First, stand up straight and squeeze/ retract your shoulder blades (scapulas) together. Tighten your bum muscles together and by taking a deep breath in, and then pull in your belly button toward your spine while you slowly breathe out for up to 30 seconds. This technique activates your foundation muscles, putting your low back spine (lumbar) in a good posture, while protecting this area. Performing this technique throughout the day will improve your posture and structural strength.

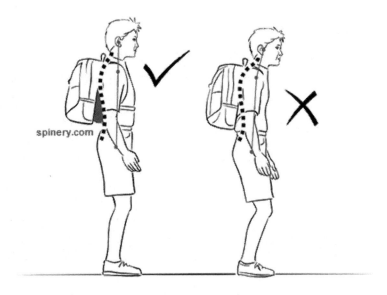

The best thing that you can do while standing is to bend (flex) your knees just slightly enough to feel your foundation muscles engage. This takes a lot of practice. Remember this, if you lock your knees, you are locking up the joints in your spine. Conversely, if you slightly flexing your knees, you are actively and consciously engaging your core muscles.

SLEEPING POSTURE:

Pressure on the back varies with sleeping position. Sleeping on the back produces the least amount of pressure, followed by sleeping on your side. Although there are copious amounts of different views on how to sleep, most experts agree that stomach sleeping is the most stressful sleeping position. So sleep on your back or side rather than your stomach whenever possible. Always use pillows under your neck and knees if you sleep on your back. Side sleepers should use pillows between their ear and bed, and between their knees to maintain spinal alignment. Your top leg should be even with your bottom leg, with both knees bent. In other words, one should sleep as if they are standing tall with a straight spine and knees slightly flexed.

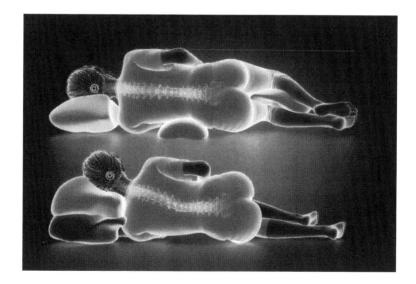

You might lose some sleep when you find out what's really inside your mattress. You and or your children spend one-third of your life in bed. You want to make sure that your mattress isn't heaving of toxic synthetic materials. Most mattresses and pillows today are made of polyurethane foam, a petroleum-based material that emits volatile organic compounds that can cause respiratory problems and skin irritation. Formaldehyde, which is used to make one of the adhesives that binds mattresses together, has been linked to asthma, allergies, and cancers. And then there are cotton pesticides and flame-retardant chemicals, which can cause cancer and nervous-system disorders.* You cannot put a price on health and here is an uncommon land mine that most people have never thought of. Search for a 'green' mattress and do your research before replacing your bedding.

*www.naturalnews.com/023246.html

*www.atsdr.cdc.gov/tfacts111.html#bookmark02

Six to eight hours per night seems to be the ideal amount of sleep for most adults, and too much or too little can have adverse effects on your health. Sleep deprivation is so ubiquitous these days that you might not even realize that you're suffering from this chronic condition. Science has now established that a sleep deficit can have serious, far-reaching effects on your health. For example, interrupted or impaired sleep can:

- dramatically weakens your immune system
- accelerate tumor growth—tumors grow two to three times faster in laboratory animals with severe sleep dysfunctions
- cause a pre-diabetic state
- seriously impair your memory
- impair your physical and mental performance
- decrease your problem-solving abilities
- increase stress-related disorders, including heart disease, ulcers, constipation and depression
- prematurely age you by interfering with your growth hormone production

Here are some tips that should improve your sleep radically:

- Sleep in complete darkness or as close to it as possible, so you don't disturb your internal clock and your pineal gland's production of melatonin and serotonin. This will help decrease your risk of cancer.
- Close your bedroom door and switch off any nightlights.
- Cover your windows with blackout shades or drapes.

- The optimal room temperature for sleep should be quite cool, between 16 to 20 °C. A room cooler or hotter than that can lead to restless sleep.
- Remove phones, TVs, digital clocks, media gadgets or any other device that produces electro-magnetic fields (EMFs). If you have Wi-Fi, put it on a timer that shuts off while you sleep. EMFs can disrupt the pineal gland and the production of melatonin and serotonin, and may have a plethora of other negative effects as well. Mattresses with metal springs may also create EMF disturbance patterns.
- Avoid before-bed snacks, particularly grains and sugars. These will raise your blood sugar and delay sleep. Later, when your blood sugar drops too low, you may wake up and be unable to fall back asleep.
- Avoid geopathic zones (Hartmann Grids). Since we sleep for approximately eight hours in the same spot, it is important to determine whether the place where we sleep (or work) is a geopathically stressed zone. Chronic health problems may eventually arise because of that. In some areas of Europe, it has long been public policy to prohibit the building of residences over water veins, fault zones or areas of geomagnetic disturbance because of the health hazards observed over many centuries in dwellings previously built on such sites.*

  * http://www.consumerhealth.org/articles/display.cfm?ID=19990303212216
- Again, avoid toxic pillows, bedding materials, and coverings.

JOINT NUTRITION

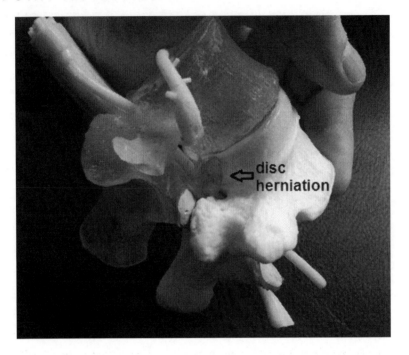

No book on bone structure would be complete without examining joint health. A joint is the connection between two bones. Joints and their surrounding structures allow you to bend your elbows, knees, hips, turn your head, and so forth.

Smooth tissue called cartilage. synovium and a lubricant called synovial fluid cushion the joints so bones do not rub together. But increasing age, injury (even sitting the wrong way or poor posture) can ultimately wear your cartilage down. This can lead to a reaction that can damage your joints and lead to arthritis.

Everyone always asks Lawrence, 'What should I take?' <u>First and</u> <u>foremost, your proper alignment is paramount for healthy</u> <u>joints.</u> Secondly, when it comes to choosing joint supplements or if you cannot get them from a natural source, here are some options:

Glucosamine is an amino acid that is naturally produced in the body. Glucosamine is the precursor to a molecule allegedly used in the formation and repair of cartilage. Treatment with glucosamine is based on the model that consumption of the ingredient may increase the rate at which new cartilage forms by providing more of the necessary building blocks. The recommended dose of glucosamine is 1500mg each day for one to two months. Continuing treatment may be considered if results are favorable.

A natural source of glucosamine and chondroitin is from animal marrow in the form of bone broth.

Chondroitin is the most abundant glycosaminoglycan in cartilage and is partly responsible for the resiliency. Chondroitin may also important in preventing the action of enzymes that destroy cartilage. The recommended dose of chondroitin is 800 mg each day for up to two months. Ongoing treatment is often continued if results are favorable and is commonly taken in conjunction with glucosamine.

Methylsulfonylmethane (MSM) is taken because some consider it may help support healthy ligaments. Some studies indicate that a high intake may help ease the symptoms of osteoarthritis and rheumatoid arthritis. The model is that the sulfur in MSM helps the body maintain healthy, flexible ligaments. MSM commonly is given as 2 to 6 g/day in 2 to 3 divided doses.

Foods that contain MSM are milk (contains 3.3 ppm of MSM), raw tomatoes (up to 0.86 milligram per liter of MSM), corn may contain as much as 0.11 milligram per liter of MSM), tea (0.3 ppm of MSM), and some say beer as well!

Egg Shell Membrane (NEM) is an all-natural joint health ingredient derived from the membrane, or inner lining, of eggshells. The eggshell membrane is then dried and milled into a powder form for supplementation and is composed of naturally occurring glycosaminoglycans, including chondroitin and hyaluronic acid, collagen, amino acids and other beneficial proteins that may be essential for joint health. Recommended dose is 500mg/day.

Hyaluronic Acid (HA) is a naturally occurring polysaccharide (carbohydrate) in the human body. It's present in large amounts in the spaces between skin cells, where it provides moisture, plumpness, firmness and suppleness to the skin. HA allegedly works by acting as a cushion and lubricant in the joints and other tissues. In addition, it might affect the way the body responds to injury. The recommended dosage for HA is not reliably established for oral supplements due to the range of different doses available and the lack of research on this. However, recommended dosages usually range from 20 to 120mg, with some recommendations as high as 200mg. Feedback on HA is that it is great for wrinkles as well!

Including foods high in hyaluronic acid may be an easy way to increase the amount of it in your body. Foods such as leafy greens, root vegetables, broths made from animal bones, skin and connective tissues are good sources. While there isn't a direct source of hyaluronic acid, red wine may help increase the amount that your body produces on its own.

ANCIENT JOINTS

Two decades ago, this author set off to explore skeletal degenerative disease in the midlands of Ireland. He joined two colleagues, both PhD's (Oxford and Cambridge University graduates) to accompany him to Ireland to assist in the study.

These three individuals started their expedition in archaeological excavation sites, where they analyzed indigenous skeletal bones dating back 200 to 600 years. Then, they approached local indigenous folks from the same region and compared their structural data to that which they had acquired from the survey of the skeletal bones of their ancestors.

Though they found no substantive indicators of chronic degeneration in the bones that were excavated, they did find some evidence of gout and psoriatic arthritis in specimens that were said to have been part of the aristocracy.

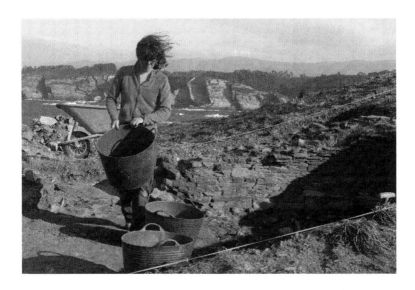

A lot of the texts and writings from this era make important distinctions between the lifestyles of the aristocracy and the lay people. According to the texts, the aristocracy led predominantly sedentary lives and consumed a diet that was comprised primarily of rich foods imported from foreign lands. The lives of peasants, on the other hand, were typified by long hours of hard labor, and their diet was comprised almost exclusively of native and in-season foods. Despite their simple diet and existence typified by physicality, Lawrence found very little evidence of chronic disease and almost no indication of arthropathy. In fact, most of the bone cortices that were analyzed had a very high mineral content compared to today's bone mineral index (BMI), and virtually no bone loss or decay was found in any of the bone structures. Lawrence wondered whether their adherence to a local, organic diet was one of the reasons for the scarcity in degenerative disease.

Lawrence was also curious about the levels of modern-day calcification in society. Calcification is the hardening of body tissues by calcium deposits or salt. The main problem with calcification is that it is insoluble, and it is like dumping sand into your engine oil. Thus, it causes inflammation; acute, chronic and arthritic pains; wrinkles; loss of hearing; arterial plaques; premature aging; oxygenation and blood flow diminishment; and bacterial and fungal infection.* *Am J Physiol Heart Circ Physiol. 287 (3): H1115–24.

A Word about Calcification....

Calcification is considered to be a contributor to nearly every condition associated with aging, such as arthritis, kidney stones, heart disease, cataracts and others. Some researchers believe that calcification is a natural by-product of aging, while other modern-day academics believe that calcification in the modern-era is caused by bacteria (nanobacteria) coursing through the system.*

*Lett Appl Microbiol. 42 (6): 549–52.

Lawrence found an abundance of calcification in the modern radiographic studies from the 'locals' that they studied along with: spinal vertebrae osteophytes, arthritis, chronic inflammation, heart disease, kidney and bladder stones, cancer, psoriasis, eczema, cataracts, heel spurs, aortic valve sclerosis and prostate stones. According to Lawrence, another overlooked pervasive challenge to the entire human body today is calcium. It is one of the most ubiquitous materials, yet the least identified culprit effecting our health today and is prevalent as a contributing factor in practically every aging condition and degenerative disease.

Thus, we should evaluate the extent to which we ingest calcium, as excessive amounts of insoluble calcium can lead to calcification. Some calcium sources, like leafy green foods, can actually be beneficial. However, other calcium sources, like calcium supplements, can be detrimental to your well-being.* We need to be careful when drinking bottled or tap water, because it is often filled with toxins and dangerous variants of minerals (like calcium). In order to ensure that your water is healthy, you can begin by filtering your water through reverse osmosis or through vorticism.

* British Medical Journal 2011; 342: d2040

Today, we live longer, but most elderly people have two to three chronic diseases that they are 'treating' perpetually. Lawrence postulates that the generations before clean water (sanitation) was a prime factor for early mortality. In other words, raw sewage in the water supply is not a good idea. Better sanitation may be the lone causative influence for life expectancy.

Another good point to think of is that if someone's modern diet during winter in the northern hemisphere consisted of many exotic and citrusy foods from the tropics, his or her blood biochemistry would change. The body thinks that its summer and so the blood thins to suit that climate and that individual may get sick. Alternatively, if someone in the tropics changed their diet to eat what Eskimos eat (blubber), his or her body may have grave difficulty cooling down. If we go to any supermarket today, we will find fruits, vegetables and meats from all over the globe. If you routinely or seasonally get sick, consider eating only eating locally (or cross-latitudinally from where you reside) and monitor the difference.

We can safely assume that our ancestors ate a raw, in-season, cross-latitudinal, local, organic diet rich in minerals and vitamins. If we consider this, perhaps that is what we should be eating as well?

EXERCISE

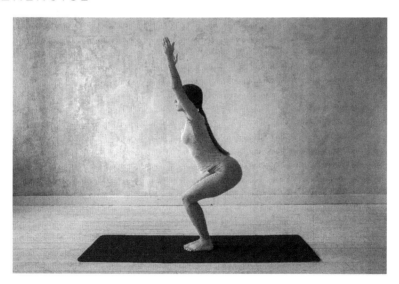

The paradox here is that the entire book is about exercising consciously in everything that you do. Exercise is simply defined as any activity that involves bodily movements which improve, develop or maintain wellness. There are various reasons why people get themselves involved in different forms of exercise. Some do it to get leaner and lose weight, reduce stress, socialize, get out in nature, and others do it to have fun. When doing any exercises, here are some considerations:

Exercise is beneficial when done properly, consciously, and when all of the foundation muscles are utilized coherently. For example, imagine going to see an orchestra where the woodwind instruments decide not to play. The sound of the music wouldn't be harmonic.

The advice we are almost always given by some 'expert' in back pain is 'exercise.' The first question that you should ask yourself is: are you exercising in a stable or unstable environment? Would you drive your car if its alignment were off? You probably wouldn't, because it would cause uneven tire wear and, ultimately, ball joint erosion.

One should exercise to develop proper movement patterns to the point that every daily activity is a conscious movement pattern in which the body is actively engaged. For example, many years ago, the author had the opportunity to watch the world's top tennis player train at UCLA. When this particular character missed a shot, he would stop and visualize his mistake at least a dozen times in his head before proceeding back to his game. The people watching stated that this behaviour was dramatic and excessive. But was it? Perhaps your exercise can be performed the same way. Strengthening your body with proper mechanics consciously over a long period of time may lead, ultimately, to the development of subconscious movement patterns in which the body is actively engaged.

Exercise should ultimately require no volition on your part. Repetitive conscious movement patterns should ultimately lead to subconscious proper harmonic activities in everything that you do from walking the dog to sitting at a lecture. And remember, exercise alone cannot undue bad posture.

"Even if people meet the current recommendation of 30 minutes of physical activity on most days each week, there may be significant adverse metabolic and health effects from prolonged sitting – the activity that dominates most people's remaining "non-exercise" waking hours."
—*N. Owen, A. Bauman, W. Brown*

So, before you jump into an exercise program, think about the primary human movement patterns described below before adding any resistance activities to an inconsistent workout. First and foremost, you need to make sure that your exercise doesn't injure you. Any exercises done improperly will break your muscles, joints and even discs down, due to the addition of resistance in the wrong places, which furthers degeneration.

One thing to keep in mind is that every muscle that directly connects to your pelvis should be considered a part of your foundation muscles. Your flexibility, strength and balance are all dependent on powerful hips. The following muscles should be connected to every exercise regimen:

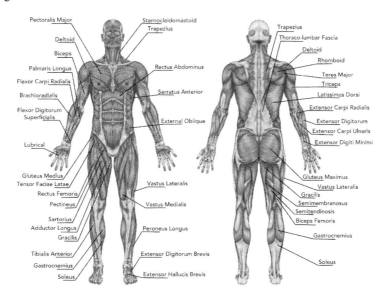

1. **The Gluteal Muscles** – These are the dynamos of your core. They cannot work independently.

2. **The Posterior Chain Muscles**: The reality is that the muscles which make up this chain are directly responsible for producing hip extension. The muscles that make up the posterior chain are as follows, with their roles stated between brackets:
- **Multifidus** (spine support)
- **Erector Spinae** (back and spinal extension)
- **Gluteal Muscles** (hip extensors, femoral rotation)
- **Hamstring Muscles** (hip extension, knee flexion)
- **Gastrocnemius or Calf** (plantar flexes ankle, knee flexion)
- **External Obliques** (back and spine support, in tandem with anterior core)

3. **The Abductors and Adductors** (outer and inner thigh muscles): They are your integrated traction system. As long as the abductor and adductor muscles are kept strong, you will have increased hip strength (by steadying the pelvic brace using a couple of the strongest muscles in your body) and stronger arches in your feet.

4. **The Abdomen and Hip Flexors:** Located in the lower portion of the spine and the top of the hip, hip flexor muscles insert into the upper middle portion of the thigh (femur). They help bend (flex) the hip and rotate the thigh externally. If these are out of balance, then the back is not working properly.

5. **The Transverse Abdominal Muscle:** A built-in bracing system. The TVA acts as a muscular girdle, stabilizing your pelvis and providing support against outside forces. It guards against repetitive physical stresses from numerous motions your body makes, such as twisting, bending, running, etc. A strong TVA will help you transfer force more proficiently through the muscles, rather than through your back and joints. This will reduce the incidence of injury caused by related stresses. When the transverse abdominis is tightened against the other muscles among this core group, the entire system becomes stronger.

So, if you are thinking of going to the gym and hiring a personal gym instructor to help you do posture correction exercise, you may need to pause for a moment. There are various exercises that do not require fancy equipment and have been shown to be effective in correcting posture if you keep **ACE** in mind. So save yourself from too much hassle and start correcting your posture with the following simple routine exercise routines if you need to go down this road:

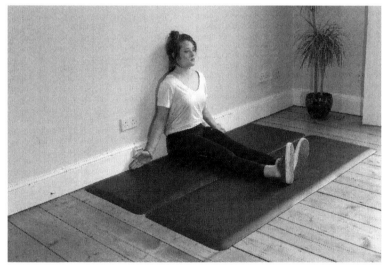

Back against the wall with your feet straight out and toes flexing back to you. Try to relax your back muscles and press your shoulders flat against the wall. Externally rotate your hands to keep your shoulders square. Hold this posture for a few minutes.

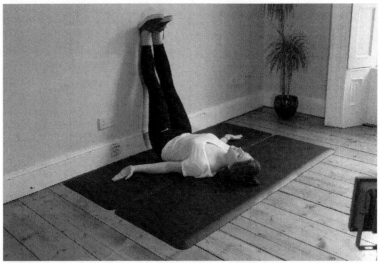

A similar variation. This time, your legs are against the wall with your feet straight out and toes flexing back to you. Try to relax your back muscles and press your shoulders flat against the wall. Externally rotate your hands to keep your shoulders square. Hold this posture for a few minutes if you can.

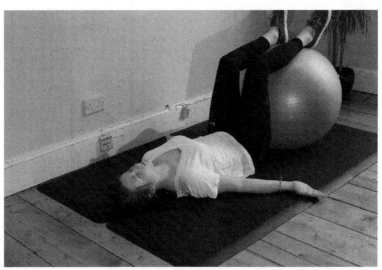

Lie down on your back, with your legs on a chair or a ball, flexed at 90 degrees with your arms just below your shoulders, and your palms facing up. Relax your lower back muscles onto the floor and hold this position for a few minutes.

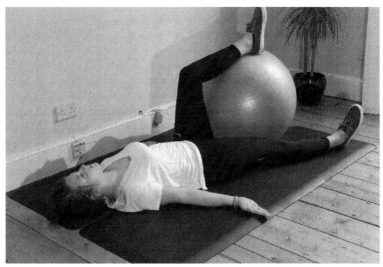

Same position as above, only this time the right leg is extended flat on the floor and the right foot is flexed at 12 o'clock. Externally rotate your hands to keep your shoulders square. Hold until your lower back muscles release.

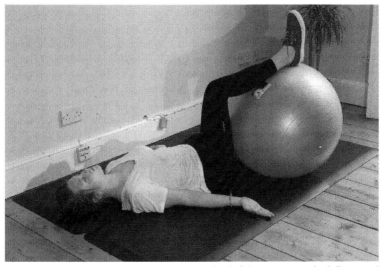

Same position as above, only this time the left leg is extended flat on the floor and the left foot is flexed at 12 o'clock. Externally rotate your hands to keep your shoulders square. Hold until your lower back muscles release.

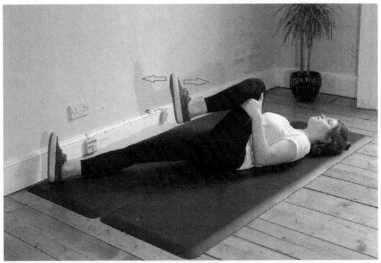

Another beneficial floor position would be to pull your knee up with the opposite leg extended and toes flexed towards the head. Now, rhythmically point and flex the ankle of the leg that you pulled up. Repeat this on the other side.

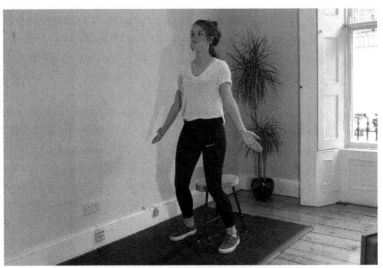

Squatting with chair. Same principle applies here as well, your weight is on your heels; ears, shoulders, hips and ankles aligned vertically; as you're squatting down, keep the bum muscles back and your head above your shoulders.

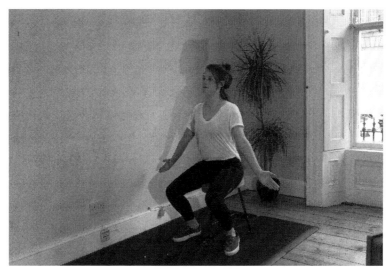

As your bum touches the chair, again, make sure that your ears, shoulders and hips are aligned vertically, with your hands externally rotated and shoulders square.

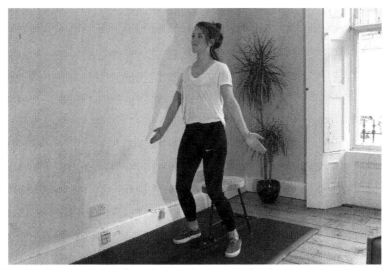

Then back up again with your weight on your heels. Engage your quads, bum, hamstrings and posterior chain muscles while relaxing your neck and shoulder muscles, and keep hands externally rotated. This exercise can easily be done at your desk throughout the day.

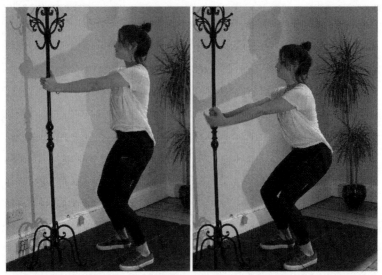

Same can be easily improvised using a pole or railing for a squatting exercise (be creative!).

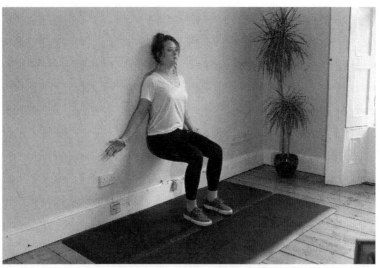

The chair squat starts with your feet shoulder-width apart and approximately a foot away from the wall. Gently put your back against the wall and slowly slide down until your knees are at 90 degrees, with your hands externally rotated, and head, shoulders, spine and bum gently pressed against the wall. See if you can ultimately work up to a few minutes.

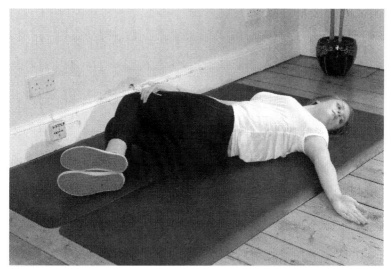

On your side, in a semi-foetal position, with knees bent, an ankle-knee-hips angle of 90 degrees, and arms out in front of you, with hands clasped and slightly below shoulder (the knees and ankles must be arranged on top of each other throughout this exercise). Now, with your hips and knees in the same position, bring your top arm across your body and let your head rotate with it. Take your bottom and place it on your knees to hold them in place. If you can, try to turn your head towards your outstretched (externally rotated) hand and relax into this position for a few minutes, and repeat on the other side.

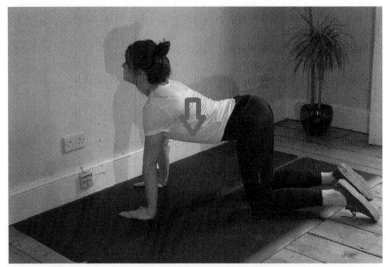

These next two exercises should be done rhythmically. Start with your head up and lower back extended.

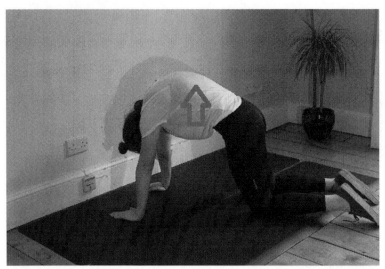

Now gently lower your head as you flex your spine. Try not to hold your breath. Keep breathing (into your stomach) while doing this exercise. Work up to a few minutes on these.

There are other more common exercises that the author recommends as well. Again, try to be actively consciously engaged while performing these:

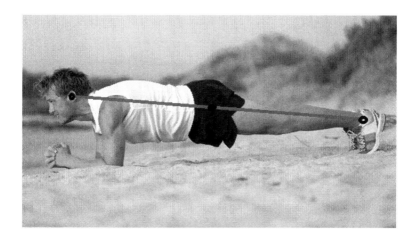

Planking – planking is a fantastic posture corrective exercise that targets the core muscles. It strengthens and stretches not only the abdominal muscles, but the shoulders and back as well. There are variations of planking depending on the specific muscles that you want to correct.

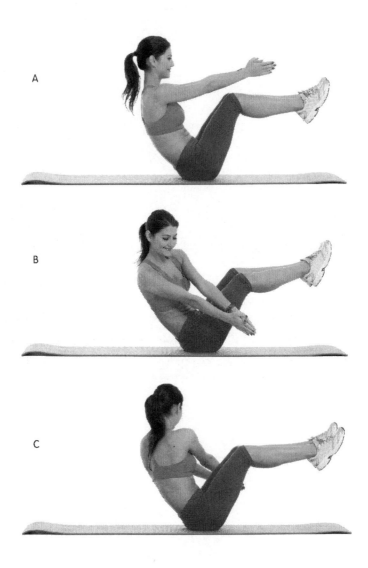

Crunch and Twist – this type of exercise is perfect for those who need to correct their oblique and abdominal muscles. This can simply be executed on a yoga mat and does not need any complex gym equipment. Do not forget to inhale and exhale repeatedly while doing the exercise to facilitate proper breathing.

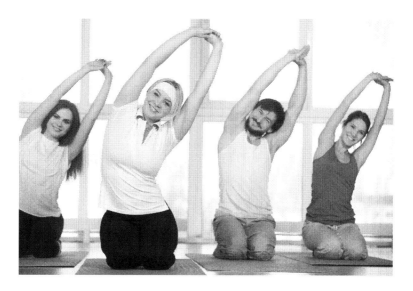

Side Bend – this exercise needs a light weight to be held on one side while bending. You may use regular dumbbells or you may improvise by using bottles filled with water. Start with lighter weights so as not to induce trauma to your muscles. This regimen corrects uneven shoulders and posture deviation, so see to it that you are doing the same number of repetitions on both sides.

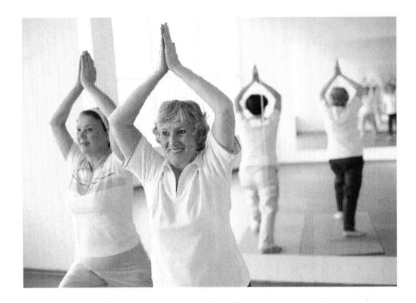

Yoga – this is a discipline-oriented exercise that does not only focus on physical but also on mental and spiritual aspects. It involves a lot of concentration and stretching procedures that hone your muscles and joints, leading to better posture. Studies show that yoga is one of the most effective posture correction exercises.

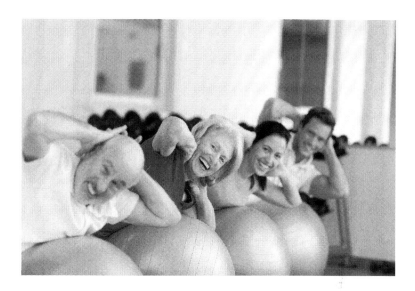

Pilates – Pilates is an exercise that involves controlled movements and a focus on consistency and precision. It helps improve the flexibility, strength and endurance of the body. It has different levels of difficulty and intensity, so it's better to know your limits in order to avoid injury. Pilates focuses on alignment, breathing and strengthening your core; that is why it is good for correcting posture.

This author would like to share a personal story of why he decided to write this book. Lawrence was finishing up his work schedule and was about to leave his clinic for the day. To his surprise, he found a group of people, all of them in their late teens, seated in his waiting room. They were all chatting away with each other. However, they were strikingly seated perfectly (Actively Consciously Engaged)!

Their spines were in perfect alignment with their knees, and, well below, the hips and foundation muscles were engaged. Lawrence didn't recognize these people at first, but then suddenly realized that they were a few of the students from the school in which his office presented postural training for one year. They just stopped by for a social visit.

After chatting with these teenagers, Lawrence was so inspired by the profound impact of working with a small group of people that he felt that maybe he should take this philosophy of conscious engagement on every level to those who want to optimally adapt to their environment. To paraphrase Shakespeare, 'the fragrance of the rose lingers on the hand that cast it'. Can you imagine what it would be like to live in a world where individuals where more consciously engaged by their own volition?

Best of luck to you in your incredible journey to absolute health. Please feel free to comment or post any queries on our website. We will keep you up to date with brilliant stories and many tips for you to acquire and preserve your active conscious engaged body.

Slainte!
Lawrence

Printed in Great Britain
by Amazon